# THE **REDOX** PROMISE

# THE **REDOX** PROMISE

## The Key to Cellular Resilience and Better Aging

**PLUS: 30 Supplements to Re-Energize Your Brain and Body**

WILLIAM A. SEEDS, MD

Published by
SSRP Institute
Madison, Ohio

ISBN 9798218448271 (print)
ISBN 9798218448288 (ebook)

Book design and production by Happenstance Type-O-Rama
Typset in Adobe Caslon Pro and Bebas Pro

First Edition

# CONTENTS



## Part 1

### The Secret to Better Aging



## Part 2

### 30 Supplements to Optimize Health and Regenerate Your Brain and Body

# Part 3

## The Three Pillars of Cellular Resilience and Healthy Aging

# INTRODUCTION

The past several years have revealed a lot about how vulnerable we are to viruses and other pathogens in our midst. Now more than ever, it's clear that understanding our cellular health and degree of cell efficiency influences the fate not only of our immune system and metabolism but also of the very quality of our lives. In this era of enormous scientific advancements happening at an increasingly faster pace, we find ourselves with an important opportunity in medical education and clinical practice to harness new research and apply it to our lives in the here and now. Indeed, my work training physicians to deepen their understanding of cellular medicine has made it clear that we have the power to understand how diseases blamed on aging can be avoided, as well as how to apply the science of cellular medicine to unlock the secrets of how to age better: not simply extending the lifespan, but promising an improved *health span.*

I've spent most of my medical career as an orthopedic surgeon, but for the past 30 years, I've focused on cellular medicine, which is redefining regenerative and functional medicine by placing the emphasis on preventative care and the ways we can integrate peptides and over-the-counter supplements to support health, well-being, and a higher quality of life as we age. Specifically, I've been researching and applying the science of peptides to optimize healing and prevent disease; this work culminated in the publication of my first book, *Peptide Protocols* (2020). More recently, I developed an educational platform and certification program for physicians to ensure that those who are interested in practicing regenerative medicine can do so with a full and accurate understanding of the science that undergirds it: cellular medicine. If we don't truly understand how cells work, produce energy, use energy, and communicate with each other, as well as how their functioning and signaling can get disrupted, then we will always be chasing our proverbial tails, spending energy and dollars on cures to diseases that could be avoided preemptively. Unlike many in the field who think of aging as a disease, I think of it as a natural slowing down of various cellular systems, which, when re-energized, can return to efficiency and function better. Indeed, my approach to cellular medicine offers physicians and patients alike a new way to think about preserving their health and maximizing healing: by targeting the body's cells, which in turn enables systems—from cardiac to respiratory to nervous and immune—to sustain their energy and cell efficiency for an improved health span. While many physicians committed to regenerative medicine want their patients to reverse aging and defeat disease by taking preventative measures, my approach takes prevention an important step further. I've systematically isolated the cellular mechanisms that affect an integral process at the heart of the aging problem: cellular redox.

*The Redox Promise* is the first book to offer powerful insights into the intricate workings of how the process of *redox* (reduction-oxidation) and maintaining its balance can offer people the energy and cell efficiency to age better. *Redox balance* refers to the equilibrium between *oxidants* (substances that cause oxidation) and *antioxidants* (substances that counteract oxidation); when this balance is disturbed, a cascade of disease-causing conditions are triggered. In the pages ahead, I will unpack the importance of redox balance, for it offers a powerful lens through which we can understand how to halt the cellular mechanisms associated with aging poorly and the diseases that can—but don't have to—develop, including heart disease, type 2 diabetes, cancer, neurodegenerative diseases, and more. These insights have the potential to revolutionize our understanding of health and disease, giving us the tools to harness the natural healing abilities of the body.

The growing interest in regenerative medicine today is truly inspiring. It's amazing for me to see my colleagues and aspiring researchers stepping into this arena with enthusiasm and curiosity, highlighting the appeal and possibilities of this field. However, along with this surge in interest comes a challenge. There are an increasing number of professionals who claim expertise in this discipline but who do not have the requisite training to target the underlying cell systems that are at the root of disease and negative aging. This is resulting in confusion due to varying levels of knowledge among these self-proclaimed authorities.

The domain of medicine as it stands today can be compared to the wilderness of the Wild West: full of opportunities as well as potential challenges and dangers. I say this with humility, as I do not proclaim myself an expert. Instead, I consider myself a lifelong learner who is devoted to exploring biology, biochemistry, quantum physics, and the underlying principles of cellular metabolism. Over the course of more than 40 years, I have tirelessly pursued knowledge in the still-burgeoning field of cellular medicine. However, every time I thought I had grasped a concept or unraveled a mechanism, I was reminded of how much remains unknown in this field and was humbled by its vastness. I share my journey—with its ups and its downs—not to boast but out of concern. It saddens me to witness individuals prematurely claiming mastery but armed with only fragments of knowledge that can be misused, harming others and posing a risk to the credibility of cellular medicine—a field that holds immense potential for revolutionizing healthcare.

The good news is that the medical field is now focused on translating the latest research in cellular metabolism and immunobiology to develop a more comprehensive and accurate understanding of how we can improve our health. I've been fortunate to be at the forefront of this drive to innovate regenerative medicine. Over a decade ago, I created Seeds Scientific Research & Performance to develop a comprehensive collection of research on cellular medicine and peptides, which enabled me to build the foundations of advanced peptide training curricula for physicians and other healthcare practitioners. My approach to cellular medicine education led me to found The International Peptide Society to provide a source of scientifically reliable information to fellow physicians. I then formed the Seeds Scientific Research & Performance (SSRP) Institute, a research-oriented consortium where physicians and other healthcare practitioners can train with me and other experts from around the world to improve their understanding of the intricacies of cellular medicine so that they can better treat their patients suffering from chronic inflammatory diseases such as heart disease, type 2 diabetes, and obesity, as well as metabolic problems, cancer, and autoimmune disorders. The SSRP is working very hard at collecting clinical data to provide an evidence-based approach to further validate treatment protocols that are already making a difference in the lives of thousands of patients.

While we have taken this knowledge of cellular medicine to prevent disease, improve performance, and change the present paradigm of aging to the point where we have increased longevity, we really have not improved the quality of life during those longevity years. In fact, we have increased the incidence of chronic disease states, with aging as the number-one risk factor. This means these are very exciting times for the field of cellular medicine.

Many books have offered helpful ways to improve health and longevity by focusing on diet and exercise, but none of them have offered a comprehensive, research-backed road map that targets cell systems and regulates overall metabolism and homeostasis. In this book, you will come to appreciate how all diseases can be traced back to a disruption in cellular balance. In my first book, *Peptide Protocols*, I shared some of this background on cellular functioning, especially as it pertains to cellular senescence and how certain peptides can counteract the deleterious effects of senescence. In this book, I take the research and its applications a step further and show how the processes of cellular redox—the reduction-oxidation cycles that provide cellular energy—are at the root of our ability to resist illness and disease *and* fight aging. And the very good news is that keeping cellular redox in balance does not have to be complicated; it's about giving the body what it needs to supply the brain and the body with proper nutrients, eliminate waste, and maintain cellular balance. This means enabling the brain to work faster and smarter and giving the body the fuel it needs so that it runs like a Tesla instead of a gas-guzzling Chevy.

My approach to cellular medicine offers a hands-on method to improve our quality of life immediately and put us on the road to healthy aging. At the cellular level, you will learn how to set up the body's cell systems to become more efficient so that internal homeostasis is maintained, and the body's cells become more resilient to epigenetic factors. In science-speak, cell efficiency promotes optimal energy metabolism; supports the immune system's ability to protect us from illness and disease; improves microbiome balance and diversity (which in my opinion are related 99.9% of the time); and, most importantly, supports cellular redox. *Cellular redox* refers to the balance between reducing agents and oxidizing agents within cells, which is essential for maintaining cellular function and preventing disease. This book recognizes the critical role that cellular redox plays in achieving optimal health, and it highlights how supplements can support this process.

This book also provides information on 30 powerful over-the-counter supplements that will strengthen the cell system. In addition, it shows how incorporating good sleep, a healthy diet, and regular exercise will maximize the impact of the supplements to balance cellular redox and energize the immune system. Therefore, this book is not just about supplements but about a comprehensive approach to health and well-being.

I treat my patients as partners in their health. I want to help them avoid medicines that can cause lifelong dependencies and other symptoms that are completely avoidable. As a physician, I empower my patients to prevent disease from happening, to access the most cutting-edge strategies in regenerative medicine, and to take charge of their health.

*The Redox Promise* is meant to guide physicians and other practitioners to apply the most up-to-date research on cellular medicine and use these evidence-backed strategies to improve the lives of their patients. I've presented the information in such a way that physicians will feel comfortable sharing it with their patients, which of course I encourage. I'm all about prevention of illness and optimizing health, but I'm also realistic: It's hard to live a perfect lifestyle . . . and indeed, that's not necessary. The body truly is intelligent, and with the redox road map, you will help your patients enhance their quality of life and stop using their energy to fight aging.

In Part 1, I will explain the importance of cellular redox and how it influences overall health and functioning. Through the lens of redox, we can appreciate how cellular homeostasis, cellular metabolism, cellular metabolic efficiency, microbiome integrity, the immune system, and modulation can be supported.

In Part 2, I provide a list of 30 supplements that target the cellular pathways that support redox balance, decrease inflammation, balance the gut's microbiome, and empower the immune system to do its job: protect our health. These supplements are over-the-counter agents that fight inflammation, support gut health, build muscle and bone, and give the immune system the energy it needs to protect against disease and negative aging.

In Part 3, I offer guidelines on how to eat, exercise, and maintain high-quality sleep so that the mechanisms of the supplements can be maximized. Together, the supplements and these lifestyle strategies will improve the necessary redox balance to age better and prevent disease. I have observed *all* of my patients benefit from these protocols and improve their energy, mental focus, and well-being, regardless of their age or background.

I am excited to share *The Redox Promise* with you and your patients. Join me on this journey as we explore the fascinating world of cellular redox and supplements and discover how everyone can enhance their overall health and vitality, now and into the future.

# The Secret to
# Better Aging



## PART 1

## A NEW MEDICAL PARADIGM THAT REDEFINES AGING

Although I am an orthopedic surgeon trained to do surgery, I've always pushed back on the idea that operating on my patients is the only way to get results for them. In fact, more than 20 years ago, I began to realize that many of my patients could achieve better health results if they did *not* have surgery. That may sound a little suspicious coming from a physician whose livelihood was largely based on both the number of surgeries I performed and their outcomes. But what I realized was that there was something wrong with a medical system that depends on waiting for disease to develop before treating symptoms and hoping for cures. Now, don't get me wrong: Medical research over the past 100 years has uncovered amazing drugs and treatments to combat devastating illnesses and diseases. But we are in a different place and time now, one that offers us the opportunity to truly prevent disease from taking root and integrates the know-how to age in a healthy way that preserves a high quality of life.

Over the last 30 years, I have focused primarily on cellular medicine, diving into the existing research, so that I could develop a keener understanding of the nuances of cell health and dysfunction. I dove into the existing research and began to do some of my own to better understand the nuances of cell health and dysfunction and how one becomes the other. The research made sense. The body's cellular systems are both supremely intelligent and adaptive, designed to protect us from a host of pathogens in our ever-changing, ever-challenging environment. These molecular pathways encompass a complicated system of cellular signaling related to homeostasis, brain functioning, metabolic health, and immune regulation, all of which interact with one another to ensure that environmental invaders such as bacteria, viruses, and other threats to our health don't get through the body's natural armor. And though the brain and body always react to such outside stressors, they are also amazingly resilient and adaptable. Indeed, the very nature of our extraordinary immune system is its many mechanisms for protection and healing. In other words, the body wants to be healthy, and preserving that health means making sure our body and brain get what they need.

This sounds simple, and it is, but there's a common obstacle to understanding how to give the body what it needs: Western medicine's reliance on drugs and intervention procedures to treat symptoms of disease. This dependence stems from an antiquated way of thinking about and applying medical advances, one that overlooks an enormous opportunity to avoid disease, preserve health, and extend a high quality of life. Indeed, most scientists and medical doctors still think of aging as a disease instead of what it is: a gradual slowing down of cellular processes. If we shift our thinking about aging to this more accurate way and seize the opportunity to re-energize our cellular systems by giving the cells what they need to stay efficient, then the so-called negative effects of aging—the digestive problems, the sleep problems, the loss of energy, the dwindling of mental focus, the memory loss, the loss of muscle and bone strength—are no longer inevitable. My approach to longevity is about aging better. I don't want to help my patients extend their lives for the sake of it; rather, I want to focus on how they can remain vital and productive and able to enjoy all of what they want to do in their so-called "second half." This is a paradigm shift based on real science and one that will reshape your patient outcomes now and into the future.

## CELLULAR REDOX: A KEY CONTRIBUTOR TO CELL EFFICIENCY

As practitioners committed to preventing and halting disease, producing better treatment outcomes when our patients do get sick, and redefining the expectations of so-called normal aging, it's important for us to incorporate recent research that points to the importance of cellular redox and its impact on how the body continues to produce and utilize energy. This vast, interconnected metabolic system is made up of more than 8,700 reactions and 16,000 metabolites. As we age, the pathways and mechanisms of this system become more vulnerable to damage, which in turn leads to loss of function and/or illness or disease. Understanding and applying the right timing and using an array of supplemental interventions, we can support the body so that it can more effectively control the excretion of toxins and arrest the buildup of other harmful metabolites. Specifically, by supporting redox—the chemical reactions that occur within cells to maintain a balance between reducing and oxidizing agents—we have a targeted method of supporting overall homeostasis, cellular efficiency, microbiome integrity, and productive immunity.

Redox homeostasis is the most important way the body achieves this multifrontal offense to control inflammation, the single most powerful cause of diseases that lead to phenotypic changes and genetic mutations. Indeed, helping the body achieve redox balance can help us age better because it

- improves mitochondrial function,

- increases cell efficiency,

- tamps down inflammation,

- mitigates oxidative stress,

- helps transport nutrients to cells,

- supports microbiome integrity,

- restores immune adaptability, and

- protects nuclear and mitochondrial DNA from epigenetic damage.

As a quick reminder, in redox, molecules gain or lose electrons, leading to changes in their oxidation state. Oxidation is the process by which a molecule loses electrons, while reduction is the process by which a molecule gains electrons. Cellular oxidation is necessary for a number of processes, including cellular respiration, the process by which cells extract energy in the form of glucose from nutrients, feeding glycolosis, the citric acid cycle (Krebs cycle), and the electron transfer system. Oxidation reactions also contribute to the breakdown of fatty acids and amino acids for energy production, two additional aspects of core cellular metabolism. These processes are crucial for providing cells with the necessary building blocks and energy to carry out various cellular and whole-organ functions.

Oxidation is also an integral part of supporting the immune system through detoxification of harmful substances within cells by converting such compounds into water-soluble forms that can be excreted by the body. Further, immune cells, such as macrophages and neutrophils, use reactive oxygen species (ROS)—the by-product of oxidation—as part of their defense mechanisms to destroy invading pathogens and protect against the development of disease. However, ROS are necessary in only moderate amounts, as they act as signaling molecules that modulate the activity of specific proteins important to cell metabolism, regulation, and immune functions such as apoptosis.

Although cellular oxidation is necessary for these important physiological processes, the human body relies on the antioxidant system to control too-high production of ROS and avoid oxidative stress that can trigger a cascade of damaging cellular conditions that upset its ability to stay in homeostasis. This is where reduction processes come into play. Antioxidants are types of reducing agents that counteract oxidative stress and prevent the slippery slope related to loss of cell efficiency, lack of nutrition to cells, and poor cell signaling. (For the purposes of this book, I will be treating antioxidants as a general type of reducing agent.) They are on the front lines, protecting cells from damage caused by ROS and free radicals by donating electrons to neutralize ROS, thereby preventing the chain reactions that lead to cellular damage. Antioxidants also help preserve the structural and functional integrity of cellular components including proteins, lipids, and DNA. Further, since mitochondria, the primary site of cellular respiration, generate ROS as by-products, antioxidants mitigate the impact of ROS on mitochondrial function, ensuring efficient energy production and preventing damage to mitochondrial DNA. Some reducing agents, such as glutathione (GSH), serve as important regulators of cellular signaling pathways. Redox-sensitive signaling molecules and transcription factors are modulated by changes in the cellular redox state, influencing processes such as cell growth, differentiation, and apoptosis. In addition, antioxidants help maintain enzymatic activities important to cellular function. Many enzymes are sensitive to changes in redox status, and their activity is regulated by the availability of reducing agents. For example, enzymes such as superoxide dismutase (SOD) and catalase act as antioxidants in a reduced state to function. Reducing agents help protect DNA from oxidative damage, which can lead to DNA strand breaks, mutations, and other forms of damage.

In this way, reducing agents are vital for maintaining redox balance within cells, protecting them from oxidative damage. An imbalance in redox status, with too many oxidizing agents and too few reducing agents, can not only undermine cell metabolism but also feed out-of-control inflammatory responses, leading to metabolic problems, disruption of microbiome integrity, mitochondrial damage, increased cellular senescence, and an overall decrease in functioning of the immune system—all of which can cause various diseases including cancer, neurodegenerative disorders, and cardiovascular disease. It's crucial that we maintain a balance between oxidizing and reducing agents while supporting the antioxidant system and maintaining cell efficiency so that ROS do not propagate. Balance is crucial.

# ANTIOXIDANTS NECESSARY FOR REDOX BALANCE

Reducing agents are substances that donate electrons or hydrogen atoms, facilitating reduction reactions in cells. At a cellular level, these agents play a crucial role in maintaining redox balance and supporting cellular efficiency. Here is a list of some common reducing agents in cells:

- Nicotinamide adenine dinucleotide (NADH): NADH is a key reducing agent involved in energy metabolism, particularly in glycolysis and the tricarboxylic acid (TCA) cycle. It donates electrons to the electron transport chain (ETC) in mitochondria during oxidative phosphorylation.

- Nicotinamide adenine dinucleotide phosphate (NADPH): NADPH, the master regulator of antioxidants, is essential for anabolic processes such as fatty acid and cholesterol synthesis, as well as for antioxidant defense. It is generated primarily through the pentose phosphate pathway.

- Glutathione (GSH): Glutathione is a tripeptide composed of glutamate, cysteine, and glycine that acts as a major cellular antioxidant. It can donate electrons to neutralize reactive oxygen species (ROS) and protect cells from oxidative damage.

- Ascorbic acid (vitamin C): Ascorbic acid is a water-soluble antioxidant that can donate electrons, helping to scavenge free radicals. It also plays a role in regenerating other antioxidants, such as vitamin E.

- Tetrahydrobiopterin (BH4): BH4 is a cofactor involved in the synthesis of neurotransmitters and the regulation of nitric oxide synthesis. It acts as a reducing agent in various enzymatic reactions for the production of neurotransmitters.

- Ubiquinol (coenzyme Q10): Ubiquinol is an electron carrier in the mitochondrial ETC. It accepts electrons from complex I and complex II and transfers them to complex III, contributing to adenosine triphosphate (ATP) production.

- Ferredoxin: Ferredoxins are iron-sulfur proteins that act as electron carriers in various cellular processes, including photosynthesis and certain redox reactions in the mitochondria.

- Dihydrolipoic acid (DHLA): DHLA is the reduced form of lipoic acid, and it acts as a cofactor for various enzymes involved in energy metabolism. It can also regenerate other antioxidants, such as vitamin C and vitamin E.

- N-acetylcysteine (NAC): NAC is a precursor to GSH and can function as a reducing agent. It is sometimes used as a supplement to support cellular antioxidant defenses.

- Flavins (e.g., flavin mononucleotide [FMN] and flavin adenine dinucleotide [FAD]): Flavins are cofactors involved in various redox reactions, particularly in the ETC and in various enzymatic processes.

These reducing agents (aka antioxidants) work in concert with other cellular processes to maintain the redox balance in cells, ensuring the proper functioning of cellular processes and protecting cells from oxidative stress.

## ENZYMATIC AND NONENZYMATIC ANTIOXIDANT SYSTEMS

Enzymatic and nonenzymatic antioxidant systems are components of the body's defense mechanisms that protect against oxidative stress, which is caused by an imbalance between the production of reactive oxygen species (ROS) and the ability of the body to neutralize ROS. Both systems play crucial roles in maintaining cellular health and preventing damage caused by oxidative stress.

**ENZYMATIC ANTIOXIDANT SYSTEMS:**

Enzymatic antioxidants are proteins that catalyze the breakdown or removal of ROS. Following are some key enzymes in this system:

- Superoxide dismutase (SOD): Converts superoxide radicals into hydrogen peroxide and oxygen

- Catalase: Breaks down hydrogen peroxide into water and oxygen

- Glutathione peroxidase: Uses glutathione to reduce hydrogen peroxide and lipid peroxides

These are some of the important enzymes that work together to neutralize different types of ROS and maintain a balanced oxidative environment within cells.

**NONENZYMATIC ANTIOXIDANT SYSTEMS:**

Nonenzymatic antioxidants are molecules that directly neutralize free radicals or enhance the activity of enzymatic antioxidants. Following are some important nonenzymatic antioxidants:

- Vitamins (e.g., vitamin C and vitamin E): Act as scavengers of free radicals and help regenerate other antioxidants

- Glutathione (GSH): A tripeptide that plays a central role in neutralizing ROS

- Melatonin: Exhibits antioxidant properties and helps protect against oxidative stress

- Coenzyme Q10 (CoQ10): Participates in electron transport and acts as a lipid-soluble antioxidant

- Polyphenols (e.g., flavonoids and resveratrol): Found in plant-based foods and have antioxidant properties

- Minerals: Examples include iron, zinc, copper, manganese, and selenium

Nonenzymatic antioxidants are essential for preventing oxidative damage in cellular structures, including lipids, proteins, and DNA. They complement the enzymatic antioxidant defenses to provide a comprehensive antioxidant network.

Both enzymatic and nonenzymatic antioxidant systems are crucial for maintaining cellular homeostasis and protecting the body from the harmful effects of oxidative stress, which is associated with various health conditions including aging, inflammation, and chronic diseases. A balanced intake of antioxidants through a diverse and nutritious diet is essential for supporting these defense mechanisms.

## OXIDATIVE STRESS

Oxidative stress and damage can cause DNA mutations, protein misfolding, lipid peroxidation, increased stress on the endoplasmic reticulum, and other cellular damage, which can undermine our ability to age better; indeed, prolonged or uncontrolled oxidative stress directly causes disease, such as type 2 diabetes, obesity, and metabolic syndrome. Reducing agents, such as enzymatic antioxidants, glutathione (GSH), and thioredoxin, help maintain cellular redox balance by neutralizing reactive oxygen species (ROS) and other oxidizing agents. In this process, reducing agents undergo oxidation themselves and convert into their oxidized forms. However, an excess of reducing agents may reduce ROS and other oxidizing agents more quickly than they can be produced, leading to a decrease in ROS levels. This decrease in ROS levels can lead to the upregulation of nicotinamide adenine dinucleotide phosphate (NADPH) oxidase, an enzyme that produces ROS in response to low ROS levels, resulting in a paradoxical increase in ROS levels. Moreover, an excess of reducing agents can also impair the function of enzymes involved in ROS detoxification, such as superoxide dismutase (SOD) and catalase, leading to the accumulation of ROS and oxidative damage. SOD converts superoxide radicals ($O^{2-}$) into hydrogen peroxide ($H_2O_2$), which is then detoxified by other enzymes such as catalase and glutathione peroxidase. Too much GSH can reduce SOD activity, leading to the accumulation of superoxide radicals and increasing oxidative stress. Further, the accumulation of superoxide radicals can lead to the formation of other ROS, which can also exacerbate oxidative stress and damage to cellular components, including proteins, lipids, and DNA, which can contribute to cellular senescence and inflammation. (Note: for this reason, I caution people against too frequent gluthione IV treatments; again, it's important to consult your healthcare professional when considering such IV treatment.)

Catalase, another enzyme involved in ROS detoxification, can be converted to an inactive form, impairing its ability to detoxify hydrogen peroxide, leading to the accumulation of hydrogen peroxide and yet more oxidative stress.

When redox balance is disrupted due to either an increase in the production of ROS and/or reactive nitrogen species (RNS) or a decrease in ROS-scavenging capacity, certain cell signaling pathways will be negatively affected. Externally, ROS and RNS can be formed by overexposure to irradiation (i.e., UV irradiation, x-ray, gamma ray), atmospheric pollutants, and chemicals; for example, exposure to metabolites of polychlorinated biphenyls (PCBs) has been shown to increase ROS production. And becoming more apparent is the increase in nanoparticles of plastics as a toxic exposure. Internally, ROS can develop within the mitochondria due to electron leakage (from complexes I and III) of the electron-transport chain.

Mitochondria and peroxisomes are also sources of ROS, whereas immune cells such as neutrophils and macrophages possess oxygen-dependent mechanisms to fight invading microorganisms. Other endogenous (i.e., internal) sources of ROS and free radicals include membrane-associated NAD(P)H oxidase, cytochrome oxidase, and xanthine oxidase. Metals such as iron and copper can also aggravate ROS production. (This occurs when the metal becomes oxidized.)

When redox is imbalanced by an overabundance of ROS, the resulting oxidative stress can also trigger post-translational changes in signaling proteins, leading to the alteration of gene expression and transcription (leading to protein misfolding). Therefore, levels of several enzymatic agents (e.g., SOD, catalase, glutathione peroxidase) and nonenzymatic antioxidants (e.g., 4-hydroxynonenal, GSH, vitamin E, vitamin C, malondialdehyde [MDA]) can be used as markers of chronic oxidative stress. For this reason, looking at oxidative stress response can help you understand and follow the pathways of redox signaling.

When under oxidative stress, excessive ROS/RNS will attack lipids, proteins, and DNA, leading to severe and irreversible oxidative damage. Lipids are most susceptible to oxidative modification. Lipid peroxidation generates lipid radicals such as MDA, which can further attack the subsequent lipid molecules and propagate as a chain reaction. A number of amino acids, such as tryptophan, tyrosine, histidine, and particularly cysteine, are direct targets of ROS. ROS-mediated protein modification can affect protein structure and function as well as protein stability. Further, cells impact protein expression in response to oxidative stress by activating G-proteins and redox-sensitive transcription factors such as Egr-1, NF-κB, and AP-1, and by activating cellular kinases such as the mitogen-activated protein kinase (MAPK).

Moderate levels of DNA damage can trigger cell cycle arrest and initiate DNA repair processes that ensure DNA integrity. In contrast, excessive damage or failure in DNA repair can induce apoptosis, indicated by an oxidative DNA marker 8-hydroxy-2-dioxyguanosine (8-OHdG), a modified nucleoside.

The final decision as to whether the cells will survive or die is the overall outcome of the integration of signals from redox-sensitive factors and other regulatory mechanisms. ROS/RNS are present in cells and tissues, determined by the balance between the rate of production versus the clearance by different antioxidant enzymes (including SOD, glutathione peroxidase, and catalase) and compounds (GSH, ascorbate, α-tocopherol, β-carotene). ROS and RNS influence the proton motive force of the electron transport chain (ETC), which determines efficient cellular metabolism and cellular immunity (see Figure 1).

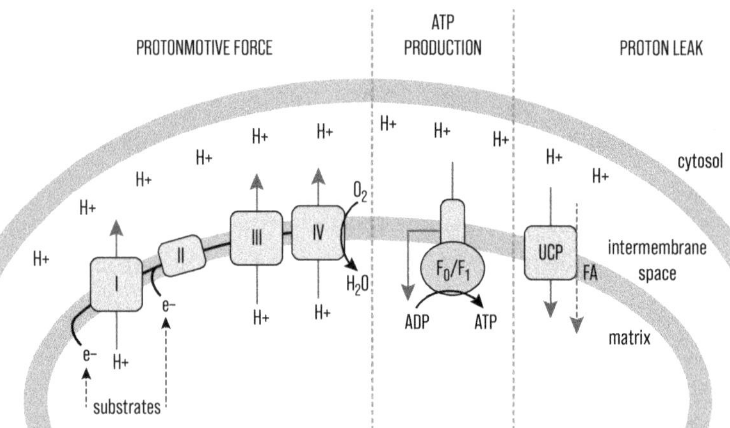


*Figure 1: Electron and proton flow determines proton motor force.*

Cells are equipped with enzymatic and nonenzymatic antioxidant systems to eliminate ROS/RNS and maintain redox homeostasis (see Figure 2).

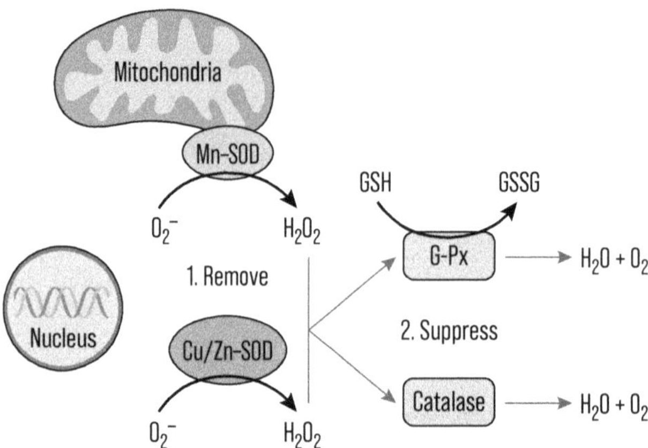


*Figure 2: Endogenous enzymatic antioxidants*

Nonenzymatic antioxidants, recognized to execute thiol-disulfide exchange reactions, also play a major role in maintaining cellular redox balance.

In addition to being a cofactor of various antioxidant enzymes, GSH, which is the most abundant peptide in cells, controls a number of functions, including scavenging of hydroxyl radicals (OH) and singlet oxygen, and regeneration of other antioxidants such as vitamins C and E and lipoic acid to their active forms. Therefore, it is essential for cells to change these oxidized proteins to their reduced forms to maintain proper function.

## CELLULAR METABOLISM AND REDOX BALANCE

The importance of energy metabolism helps us to further understand the importance of redox balance. In particular, carbohydrate, protein, and fat metabolism each play a role in maintaining redox homeostasis.

Carbohydrates undergo glycolysis, a metabolic pathway that breaks down glucose into two molecules of pyruvate. This process results in the production of two molecules of adenosine triphosphate (ATP) through substrate-level phosphorylation, where a phosphate group is transferred from a phosphorylated intermediate to adenine dinucleotide phosphate (ADP) to produce ATP. In addition to ATP, reducing equivalents such as nicotinamide adenine dinucleotide (NADH) and nicotinamide adenine dinucleotide phosphate (NADPH) are also produced during glycolysis.

Specifically, two ATP molecules are produced for each glucose molecule consumed by glycolysis, making it an important energy-yielding pathway in the cell. (See the next section for more on the progression of glycolysis in mitochondria in relation to cellular respiration.)

NADPH is also generated through an alternative pathway called the *pentose phosphate pathway* (PPP), which is an important source of reducing equivalents for biosynthetic reactions such as fatty acid synthesis and nucleotide synthesis. The PPP generates NADPH by converting glucose-6-phosphate into ribulose-5-phosphate, a reaction that is catalyzed by the enzyme glucose-6-phosphate dehydrogenase. The main reducing agent, glutathione, is kept in its reduced state by NADPH, which in turn helps to keep superoxide dismutase (SOD) and catalase in their reduced state.

NADPH plays a crucial role in activating the antioxidant system by providing reducing equivalents to maintain the levels of glutathione (GSH) in the reduced state. GSH is an important antioxidant that protects the cell against oxidative damage by scavenging reactive oxygen species (ROS). The active form of GSH, known as reduced GSH, is maintained by the enzyme glutathione reductase, which uses NADPH as a source of reducing equivalents.

The reaction catalyzed by glutathione reductase involves the reduction of oxidized glutathione (GSSG) to GSH, which requires the transfer of electrons from NADPH to GSSG (see Figure 3). This reaction helps to maintain levels of GSH in the reduced state, which is important for the antioxidant function of GSH. In addition to providing reducing equivalents for glutathione reductase, NADPH is also required for the activity of other antioxidant enzymes, such as superoxide dismutase (SOD) and catalase. SOD converts superoxide radicals into hydrogen peroxide and catalase converts hydrogen peroxide into water and oxygen. Both SOD and catalase require NADPH for their activity. All of these steps take place in the cytoplasm.

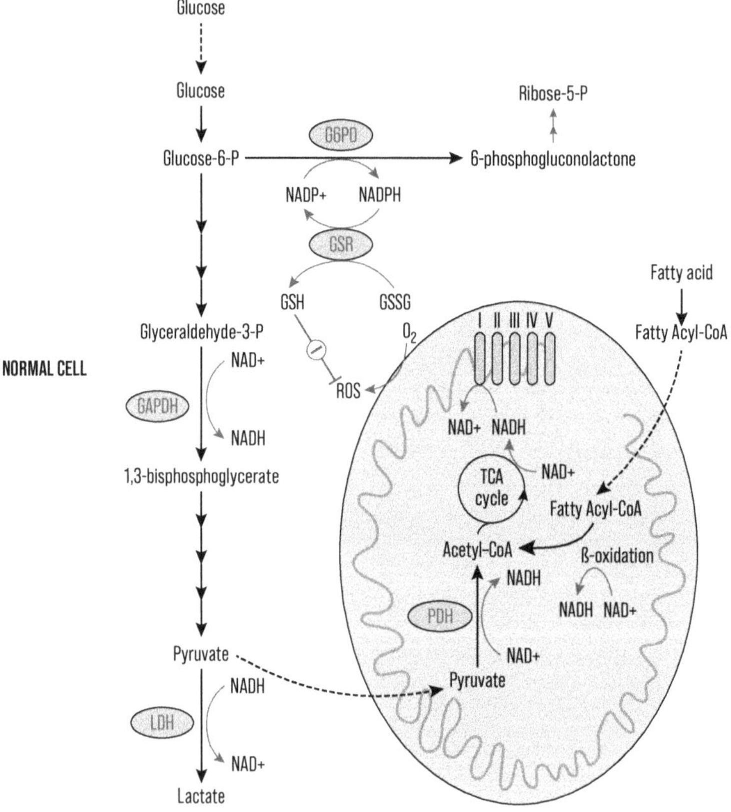


*Figure 3: Normal cell metabolism*

Dietary fats are broken down into fatty acids and glycerol in the small intestine and are transported to the liver where they undergo beta-oxidation, a process that converts fatty acids into acetyl coenzyme A (acetyl-CoA), which enters the citric acid cycle to produce reducing equivalents such as NADH and FADH2.

In addition, the glycerol component of dietary fats can enter the glycolytic pathway to produce NADH. Glycerol is a three-carbon molecule that can be derived from the breakdown of triglycerides in adipose tissue or from dietary fat intake. In the liver, glycerol is converted into glycerol-3-phosphate, which enters the glycolytic pathway as an intermediate, where it can be converted into pyruvate.

During the conversion of glycerol to pyruvate, a series of enzymatic reactions occur that result in the production of ATP, NADH, and pyruvate. The NADH produced during this process can enter the electron transport chain (ETC) in the mitochondria to generate more ATP.

The NADH and FADH2 produced during the metabolism of dietary fats are then used by the ETC in the mitochondria to generate ATP, the primary source of energy for the cell. Ingested proteins are broken down into amino acids, which in turn go through their own steps to synthesize proteins from both nonessential amino acids (made by the body) and nine essential amino acids the body needs to consume in order to produce NADH, NADPH, and ATP. Proteins are broken down into their constituent amino acids during digestion, which can then enter different metabolic pathways in the body.

Amino acids can be used for energy production or biosynthesis of new proteins, or they can be converted into other metabolic intermediates. The oxidation of amino acids produces a variety of reducing agents, including NADH, FADH2, and NADPH. The specific redox agents produced depend on the amino acid and the pathway in which it is catabolized. For example, the catabolism of the amino acid leucine produces acetyl-CoA and acetoacetate, which can enter the citric acid cycle to generate reducing equivalents such as NADH and FADH2. The catabolism of the amino acid glutamate produces alpha-ketoglutarate, which also enters the citric acid cycle to generate NADH and FADH2.

# A CLOSER LOOK AT THE ROLE OF NAD PATHWAYS

The nicotinamide adenine dinucleotide (NAD+)/reduced NAD+ (NADH) and NADP+/reduced NADP+ (NADPH) redox couples are essential for maintaining cellular redox homeostasis and for modulating numerous biological events, including cellular metabolism. A deficiency or imbalance of these two redox couples has been associated with many pathological disorders; focusing on redox stress (oxidative and reductive stress) has underscored the significance of changes in the ratios of NAD+ to NADP+. Ideal ratios are an improved increase in the ratio of NAD to NADH and a decrease in the ratio of NAP to NADPH, indicating more NAD+ (oxidizing agent) and NADPH (reducing agent) as a cofactor for improved cellular metabolism and immune cell modulation.

It is critical to understand how cells maintain the steady levels of these redox couple pools to ensure their normal function and simultaneously avoid inducing redox stress. In addition, it is essential to understand how enzymes that utilize NAD(H) and NADP(H) interact with other signaling pathways, such as those regulated by hypoxia-inducing factor 1-alpha (HIF-1 alpha), to maintain cellular redox homeostasis and energy metabolism. This is a normal muscle stress response during exercise when depleted of oxygen; NADPH oxidase becomes activated and influences HIP 1-alpha to stimulate glucose uptake by muscles through GLUT-4 receptor activation and improves insulin secretion from pancreatic beta cells.

The NAD(H) and NADP(H) redox couples serve as cofactors and/or substrates for many enzymes to maintain cellular redox homeostasis and energy metabolism. A deficiency or imbalance in cellular NAD(H) and NADP(H) levels aggravates cellular redox status and undermines metabolic homeostasis, triggering redox stress, energy stress, and eventually disease states. Thus, maintaining cellular NAD(H) and NADP(H) balance is critical for cellular function.

NAD+ is synthesized by three pathways: the de novo pathway, the Preiss–Handler pathway, and the salvage pathway. In addition to their crucial roles in maintaining cellular redox state, the NAD(H) and NADP(H) redox couples are also critical regulators of cellular metabolism. Typically, NAD+ is necessary for glycolysis and for the biosynthesis of nucleotides and amino acids; NADH provides electrons for mitochondrial oxidative phosphorylation and adenosine triphosphate (ATP) production. NADP+ supports the pentose phosphate pathway (PPP) to generate NADPH that is indispensable for reductive biosynthesis of nucleotides, amino acids, and lipids (see Figure 4).

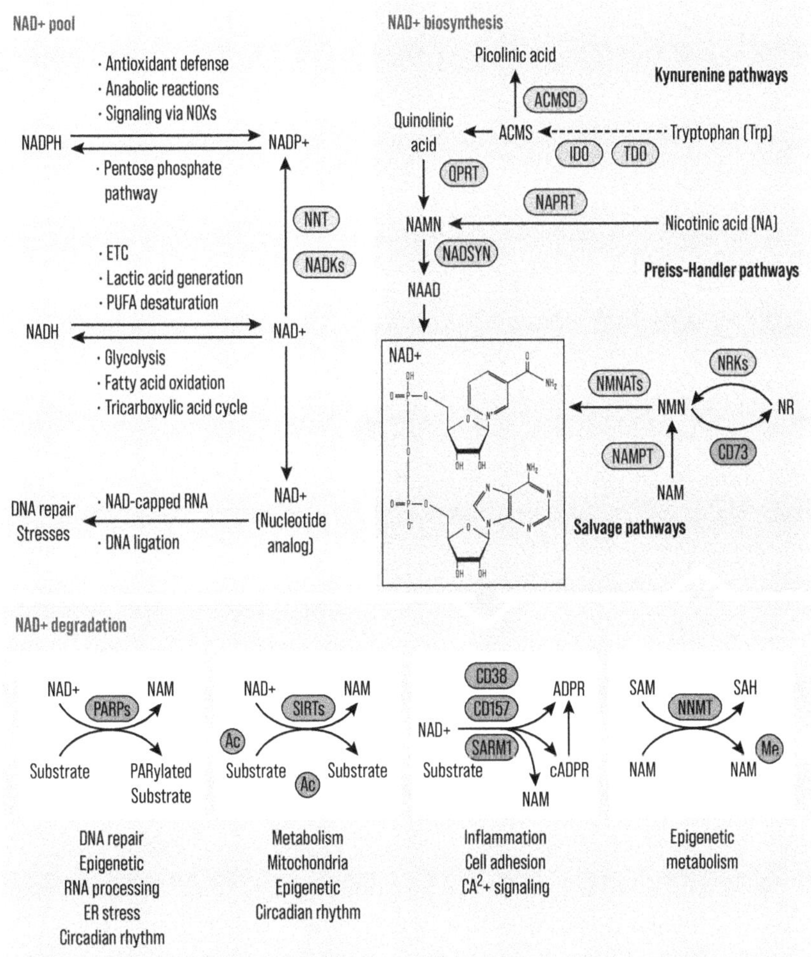


Source: Xie, N., Zhang, L., Gao, W., Huang, C., Huber, P. E., Zhou, X., Li, C., Shen, G., & Zou, B. (2020). NAD+ metabolism: pathophysiologic mechanisms and therapeutic potential. *Signal Transduction and Targeted Therapy*, 5(1), 227. https://doi.org/10.1038/s41392-020-00311-7

*Figure 4: NAD+ pathways*

The oxidized electron carriers in the mitochondrial electron transport chain (ETC) include flavin mononucleotide (FMN; complex I); flavin adenine dinucleotide (FAD; complex II); coenzyme Q (CoQ) and cytochrome b (complex III); and cytochrome c and cytochrome a/a3 (complex IV). These carriers have a higher affinity for electrons and are in their oxidized state when they accept electrons from other electron donors such as NADH or FADH2. As electrons are transferred through the ETC, these carriers become reduced and carry the electrons to the next electron acceptor in the chain (see Figure 5).

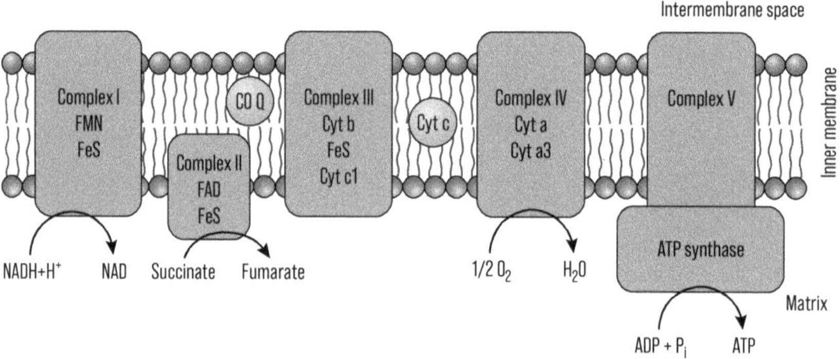


*Figure 5: Enzyme complexes of the electron transport chain*

Oxidized electron carriers are fundamental factors in how cells extract and use energy, particularly in their role in oxidative phosphorylation, a critical part of cellular respiration. Oxidative phosphorylation, which occurs in the mitochondrial inner membrane, is where the NADH and FADH2 electron carriers come in to donate their electrons to the ETC and set off a series of proteins and other molecules (including FMN,

FAD, CoQ, and cytochromes) that accept and pass along electrons in a controlled manner. In their oxidized state, these carriers have a high affinity for electrons, meaning they readily accept electrons from NADH and FADH2. As they accept electrons, they become reduced. They then pass the electrons to the next carrier in the chain and return to their oxidized state, ready to accept more electrons. This series of redox reactions creates an energy gradient used to drive the synthesis of ATP.

Keep in mind that cellular respiration, the process by which cells generate ATP (the energy currency of cells), has three primary stages: glycolysis, the Krebs cycle (also called the citric acid cycle), and oxidative phosphorylation. The first two stages occur in the cytoplasm and mitochondria matrix, respectively, and lead to the generation of NADH and FADH2. These two molecules are high-energy electron carriers. Oxygen acts as the final electron acceptor in the chain, combining with the electrons and protons (hydrogen ions) to form water. This is crucial because it maintains the flow of electrons through the ETC. This mechanism maintains the cell redox balance, ensuring that cells can generate energy efficiently.

## HOW EXERCISE IMPROVES REDOX BALANCE

A helpful way to understand redox in action is to consider the role it plays in physical exercise. During aerobic exercise, oxygen is used to break down glucose and fatty acids, releasing energy in the form of adenosine triphosphate (ATP). This process produces nicotinamide adenine dinucleotide (NADH), which is a reduced form of NAD+. During resistance exercise, ATP is used to contract muscles, a process that produces NAD+, which is an oxidized form of NADH. The overall effect of exercise increases the ratio of NAD+ to NADH, which not only helps to increase energy production but also improves redox balance.

The specific changes in NAD+ and NADH that occur during aerobic exercise are as follows: NAD+ is reduced to NADH, which is then used to produce energy. During resistance exercise, NAD+ is oxidized to produce energy. However, this association between resistance exercise and the production of ATP is both an oversimplification and a common and misleading interpretation of what's really going on. Resistance exercise, such as weight lifting, leads to muscle contraction. The energy for this contraction is powered by ATP. As we exert our muscles, they require more energy, which leads to an increased demand for ATP. This ATP is primarily produced in mitochondria through a process called oxidative phosphorylation (through the electron transport system), but also via anaerobic glycolysis, especially during high-intensity workouts. During such workouts, minimal glucose enters the mitochondria; instead, glycolosis produces the majority of NAD from conversion of pyruvate to lactate in order for glycolosis to continue to make ATP.

While ATP breakdown and NAD+ production both occur during resistance exercise, they are not directly linked. During resistance exercise, or any other physical activity, the demand for energy increases in the body, particularly in muscle cells. ATP is the main source of energy for most cellular processes, and it's broken down into adenosine diphosphate (ADP) and inorganic phosphate to release energy that can be used by the cells. This breakdown of ATP doesn't directly lead to the production of NAD+.

NAD+, on the other hand, is a coenzyme that's vital for redox reactions in the cell. It exists in two forms: an oxidized form (NAD+) and a reduced form (NADH). During cellular respiration (glycolysis, citric acid cycle, and oxidative phosphorylation), NAD+ accepts electrons (along with a proton), becoming NADH.

Resistance exercise can lead to an increase in the ratio of NAD+ to NADH, but not directly due to the breakdown of ATP. Instead, it's due to processes such as oxidative phosphorylation, where NADH donates its electrons to the electron transport chain (ETC) and is thereby converted back to NAD+, and the lactate production pathway under anaerobic conditions. During oxidative phosphorylation, the electrons are transferred from NADH and FADH2 (another coenzyme) to oxygen via a series of protein complexes in the inner mitochondrial membrane (the ETC). The energy from these electron transfers is used to pump protons across the inner mitochondrial membrane, creating a proton gradient. The flow of these protons back across the membrane drives ATP synthesis. In the process, NADH is oxidized back to NAD+. In anaerobic glycolysis, glucose is converted to pyruvate, generating ATP and NADH in the process. This occurs in the cytoplasm; it takes two ATP molecules to start the process of glycolosis, eventually producing four ATP (with a net gain of two ATP per cycle of glycolosis). However, under anaerobic conditions, the pyruvate is then converted to lactate, and in this step, the NADH is used to reduce pyruvate, regenerating NAD+.

So, in both energy-generating pathways, NADH is used and converted back to NAD+. This leads to a decrease in the NADH concentration and an increase in the NAD+ concentration, thereby increasing the ratio of NAD+ to NADH.

Moreover, resistance exercise stimulates the production of certain proteins and signaling molecules, such as AMP-activated protein kinase (AMPK) and sirtuins. These molecules can upregulate the expression of nicotinamide phosphoribosyltransferase (NAMPT), the rate-limiting enzyme in the salvage pathway of NAD+ synthesis, leading to an increased total pool of NAD+ and thereby contributing to an increased ratio of NAD+ to NADH.

However, it's important to note that the actual effect on the ratio of NAD+ to NADH can depend on several factors, including the intensity and duration of the exercise and the individual's fitness level and diet. It's also worth mentioning that the redox state of a cell (including the ratio of NAD+ to NADH) is tightly regulated, as it's critical for maintaining normal cellular function.

So, while both ATP breakdown and NAD+ production occur during resistance exercise, they are parts of different but interconnected metabolic processes. The interplay of various molecular pathways, including the ratio of NAD+ to NADH, SIRT1 activation, AMPK signaling, and the activation of antioxidant response elements (AREs), plays a role in the regulation of antioxidant gene expression.

An increased ratio of NAD+ to NADH favors the activation of enzymes that are dependent on NAD+, such as SIRT1 (a deacetylase enzyme that is a member of the sirtuin family). An enhanced ratio of NAD+ to NADH activates SIRT1, which has various functions, including the deacetylation of transcriptional coactivator PGC-1alpha (peroxisome proliferator-activated receptor gamma coactivator 1-alpha). This is an important step where PGC-1alpha has to be made available through SIRT-1 deactyalation (which happens in the cytoplasm); once PGC-1alpha is phosphorylated by AMPK, it can enter the nucleus to signal beneficial cellular changes. Phosphorylated PGC-1alpha and NRF-2, a transcription factor, bind to AREs located in the promoter regions of antioxidant genes. This binding activates the transcription of various antioxidant genes, including those encoding enzymes such as glutathione peroxidase, superoxide dismutase (SOD), catalase, heme oxygenase-1 (HO-1), and others. These antioxidants help neutralize reactive oxygen species (ROS) and reduce oxidative stress.

In this way, these pathways represent a coordinated regulation of multiple factors involved in antioxidant defense. This regulation demonstrates how an improved ratio of NAD+ to NADH, SIRT1 activation, AMPK signaling, and the activation of AREs can collectively promote the expression of antioxidant genes, leading to increased antioxidant production and protection against oxidative stress. It's important to note that the specific details of these molecular interactions and their regulation may vary depending on cell type, context, and physiological conditions. This is the beginning of gaining a better understanding of the mechanisms involved in antioxidant gene transcription, the complicated but important way of understanding the effects of different types of exercise, and its significance in maintaining cellular redox (see Figure 6).

## THE CRUCIAL ROLE OF MICROBIOME BALANCE

Lately, there has been a lot of talk about how to protect our microbiome. But there are still a lot of misconceptions about how to build a healthy gut, the primary function of which is to maintain a diverse, healthy microbiome by producing metabolites essential for efficient and flexible cellular metabolism. Indeed, the central job of our gut microbiome is to help us digest macronutrients, protect against pathogen invasion, and produce metabolites that are beneficial for cellular metabolism and our immune system, and also to help maintain cellular redox.

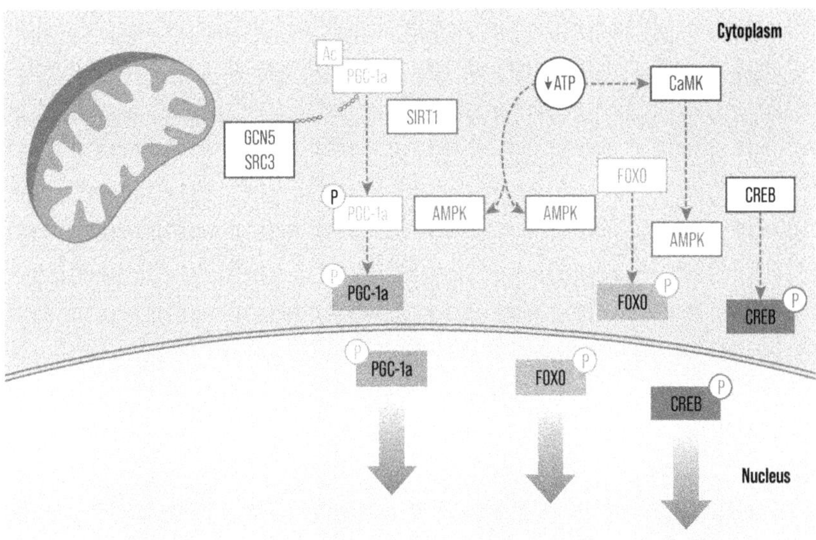




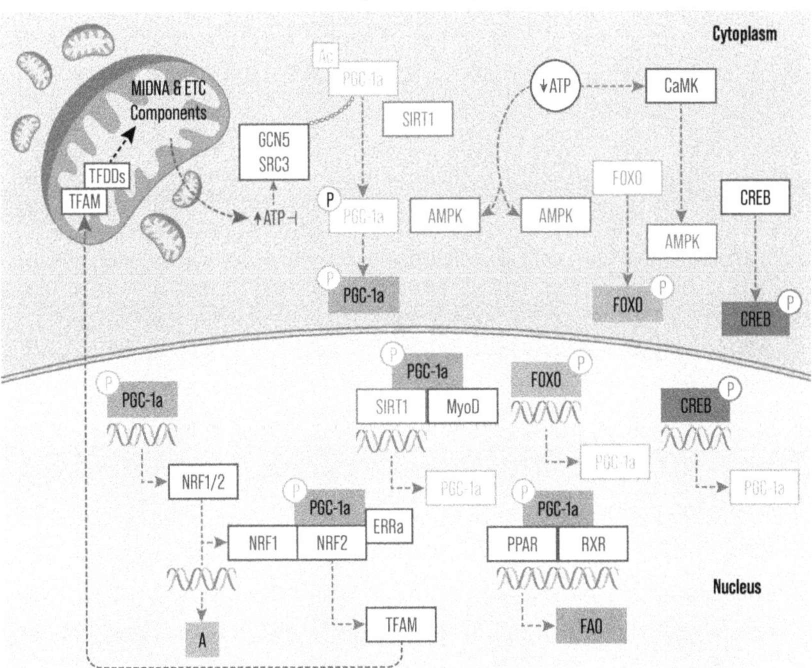


*Figure 6: Examples of PGC–1alpha from cytoplasm to nucleus and its transcription*

There has also been a lot of talk about *dysbiosis*, a term that's thrown around and often misused. Dysbiosis is the primary marker of a gut that is out of whack. It's simply a loss of real estate owned by good bacteria and a gain of opportunistic or bad bacteria (real estate) in the gut that sets the stage for loss of efficient cell metabolism and dysregulation of the immune system. It starts with loss of self-tolerance, the immune system's ability to keep good and bad bacteria in a healthy balance so that the immune system doesn't overreact. Redox balance supports the immune system in this way by keeping oxygen out of the cell so that dysbiosis, for instance, does not develop.

What does this boil down to? When the gut is overrun by bad bacteria or has too few good bacteria, the lining of the gastrointestinal (GI) tract becomes inflamed and vulnerable to undermining self-tolerance and triggering immune dysregulation. The reason dysbiosis is getting so much attention is its association with chronic diseases such as neurodegenerative diseases, heart disease, inflammatory arthropathies, Chron's disease, ulcerative colitis, irritable bowel disease (IBD), obesity, diabetes, and its increasing appearance in many immune diseases. However, the most important takeaway for general health is that dysbiosis leads to or is consistent with chronic inflammation, the root cause of most diseases and cellular senescence. For example, just as obesity leads to chronic low-grade inflammation from abnormal hypertrophied adipocytes, immune cells with polarized macrophages in the fat chronically signal pro-inflammatory mediators.

At the cellular level, dysbiosis stems from a loss of the colonic cell utilizing oxygen from the blood to effectively produce the balanced redox ratios of NAD to NADH, NADP to NADPH, acetyl coenzyme A (acetyl-CoA) to CoA, and adenine dinucleotide phosphate (ADP) to adenosine triphosphate (ATP). This can start very early in a person's life if they do not balance the macronutrients that maintain a balance of acids (proteins) with bases (vegetables and fruit); without this balance, alterations in the cellular pH can add up over time, leading to an increase in net acid load. Chronic or long-standing pH imbalance creates a maladaptive response of protein degradation, increasing the breakdown of amino acids such as glutamine from muscle to the kidney, where the acid is excreted as ammonia in the urine to decrease the acidic pH burden. This process of maintaining homeostatic acid–base mechanisms is called acidosis-induced proteolysis. A continued increase in acid over time leads to mitochondrial dysfunction, loss of cellular efficiency of colonic cell metabolism, and propagation of an altered microbiome that becomes unbalanced between good and bad bugs, leading to continued dysbiosis, sarcopenia, and eventual osteopenia.

The relationship between microbiome imbalance and redox imbalance is complex, but important to keep in mind. For instance, we know that the microbes in the gut play a crucial role in the metabolism of macronutrients and the production of microbes that can influence the redox status of the host. Gut microbes ferment dietary fibers to produce short-chain fatty acids (SCFAs), such as butyrate. SCFAs are nutrients for the cell and can lead to antioxidant production. When negative changes in the composition of the microbiome occur, SCFA production is compromised, and consequently, redox status is undermined. Further, since dysbiosis causes an increase in inflammation and promotes an overproduction of reactive oxygen species (ROS), it will also contribute to oxidative stress. Elevated oxidative stress can negatively impact the gut microbiota. Some gut microbes have the ability to produce ROS as part of their normal metabolic processes. While these ROS can contribute to the defense against other microorganisms, an overproduction can lead to oxidative stress in the host and impact the overall integrity of the gut—a vicious circle. Disruption of the gut barrier can then lead to an increase in the translocation of microbial products into the bloodstream as a result of loss of immune tolerance, thereby triggering inflammatory responses that exacerbate redox imbalance. The gut microbiome can also influence the expression and activity of host antioxidant enzymes and impact the host's ability to counteract oxidative stress through its antioxidant defenses. In addition, microbial products, such as lipopolysaccharides (LPS) from certain bacteria, can interact with host cells and induce inflammatory responses. These LPSs trigger toll-like receptor responses that lead to proinflammatory changes. Fortunately, and as you will see in the upcoming sections, we do have a number of simple yet powerful supplements and strategies to bring the gut's microbiome back into balance by reducing acidity, increasing alkalinity, and improving the protective effects of cellular redox.

A healthy microbiome is one that maintains optimal colonic cells that efficiently utilize maximal oxygen-producing NAD, NADPH, and ATP. A healthy pH is one that maintains a good ratio of acidity (proteins) to alkalinity (fruits and vegetables). The supplements and other lifestyle factors discussed in this book will help you and your patients maintain cellular pH balance and enhance the diversity of the gut microbiome, enabling the body to more effectively fight illness and disease and age better.

## HOW IMMUNE MODULATION SUPPORTS CELL EFFICIENCY

The immune system is a complex web of interacting cellular networks designed to protect us against invaders (threats or pathogens) both inside and outside the body and is integral to maintaining cellular redox and overall cellular homeostasis. In a general way, we know that anytime one part of the body is weak, other parts of the body are affected. As a result, the cells of the body rally and direct energy to any area where help is most urgently needed. When this happens, cell efficiency is stressed.

The body's immune response, which is made up of a complex interplay of biochemical, metabolic, and cellular reactions, is preprogrammed to fight against pathogens such as viruses and bacteria. It's the job of the *innate immune system* to be the first responder, sending out several signals to attack any kind of pathogen. This frontline defense releases gamma-delta T cells that act like an alarm system, alerting a series of reactions to be initiated.

Once this cycle is activated, the innate immune system is enhanced by natural killer cells, macrophages, neutrophils, monocytes, and dendritic cells. These cells recognize pathogens through pattern recognition receptors (PRRs) that detect pathogen-associated molecular patterns (PAMPs). Further innate responses will assist the adaptive immune arm, leading to TReg cells directing further macrophages, and dendritic cells to present antigens to help T cells and B cells of the adaptive immune system. B cells of the adaptive immune system produce antibodies that neutralize invaders and further activate macrophages and other T cells to engulf or neutralize the virus or other pathogens. There are other mechanisms at work as well that enable the two immune systems to continue to interact efficiently.

Think of the two systems in this way. First, the innate system is on the front line and turns on the invaders with a series of bows and arrows, pushing a virus into retreat mode. Next, the adaptive immune response comes in with its antibodies like an army of Pac-Man characters, gobbling up the weak, retreating invaders.

In this way, these two immune systems modulate each other as well as work together to fight off any disease or infection. Modulation is crucial for innate and adaptive immune functions; supercharging the immune system is not right. It's about giving the system what it needs to keep modulating and adapting. This is why "boosting" one's immune system is so erroneous. If one is compromised, it will trigger the other to work harder. If one is in hyperactive mode and overworking, the other will begin to dampen its response. While the two are usually in a give-and-take exchange, sometimes this exchange becomes dysregulated, resulting in further problems including respiratory distress, blood clots, stroke, neurological symptoms, and the exacerbation of some autoimmune disorders such as lupus or rheumatoid arthritis.

The key is to give our cells the best possible opportunity to stay efficient and in a state in which they can intelligently control their fate of better DNA repair, autophagy, mitophagy, and cellular apoptosis. Again, keep in mind the importance of striving for cell efficiency: So much of our overall health depends upon our body's cells being able to get optimal nutrition, which in turn leads to the production of NAD+, NADPH, adenosine triphosphate (ATP), and acetyl coenzyme A (acetyl-CoA) for energy, and utilization of those energy sources to stay active and growing. When this cell cycle gets depleted—from either poor sources of nutrition or an immune response that is diverting nutrition or interrupting energy production or utilization—the cells can become senescent, which is the hallmark of all sorts of inflammation and downstream diseases.

Keeping the innate and adaptive immune systems working in tandem requires that we feed our cells optimally. This is why nutrition, exercise, high-quality sleep, and other interventions are so important: They give the immune systems' cells not just adequate sources of energy, but preferable nutrition.

The immune system is intended to preserve homeostasis by combatting any internal (endogenous) or external (exogenous) stressors, toxins, or other agents that upset its capacity and efficiency for managing allostatic load (the cumulative effect of wear and tear from chronic exposure to environmental stress). For example, a preexisting condition such as diabetes, heart disease, or chronic obstructive pulmonary disease (COPD) has already increased the allostatic load of both the innate and adaptive immune systems, and therefore, all protective or defensive capabilities have become overtaxed and downregulated, including the cascading effect of overall cell inefficiency and loss of metabolic flexibility.

Again, cellular redox directly influences and indirectly regulates immune modulation. Metabolic flexibility enables the inherent intelligence of cells to regulate cellular redox and influence positive epigenetic determinants for a beneficial cell phenotype. Our best defense against any pathogen is an offense. We're not just talking about viruses and bacteria—we're also talking about allostatic stressors that undermine the microbiome, cell signaling, and other basic cell functioning. The human body is supremely intelligent and learns quickly. If we give our body the right information, it can and will do the job it's designed to do.

## THE IMMUNE SYSTEM AND REDOX BALANCE

The immune system relies on redox signaling and regulation to function properly and enhance healthy aging. Specifically, redox supports the antioxidant system. Antioxidants such as glutathione (GSH) and vitamins C and E, and enzymes such as superoxide dismutase (SOD), play a key role in neutralizing reactive oxygen species (ROS). These antioxidants help prevent oxidative damage to immune cells, ensuring their optimal functioning.

Proper redox signaling activates immune cell differentiation and communication, as well as the regulation of processes such as phagocytosis, cytokine production, and immune cell migration. Redox balance is essential for the proper execution of phagocytosis, a critical immune response in which immune cells such as macrophages and neutrophils engulf and digest foreign particles, including pathogens. Redox balance also influences the proliferation and differentiation of immune cells. ROS can act as signaling molecules in pathways that regulate the growth and differentiation of immune cells, ensuring an appropriate immune response. Redox signaling is involved in regulating apoptosis, a process that eliminates damaged or infected cells. Proper redox balance ensures the controlled activation of apoptotic pathways, preventing the survival of damaged cells that could contribute to chronic inflammation or autoimmune reactions.

## THE INNATE AND ADAPTIVE IMMUNE SYSTEMS

The innate immune system is made up of various components, including physical barriers (e.g., the skin, epithelial and mucous membranes and mucus); anatomical barriers; epithelial and phagocytic cell enzymes (e.g., lysozyme), phagocytes (neutrophils, monocytes, macrophages), and inflammation-related serum proteins (e.g., C-reactive protein and lectins); and antimicrobial peptides (including defensins and cathelicidin). The innate system also sends signals to toll-like receptors, which in turn release cytokines and inflammatory mediators (e.g., macrophages, mast cells, and natural-killer cells).

These mechanisms create a cascade of signaling events to prevent infection, eliminate invader pathogens, and then *turn on* the acquired immune response.

The adaptive or acquired immune system occurs in conjunction with the innate immune system, and ideally is responding to signals from the innate system in an ongoing way. Like the innate response, the adaptive response is designed to protect against further infection. It is also responsible for turning down the proinflammatory response of the innate arm. This signaling is typically regulated by TReg and BReg cells. The adaptive immune response relies principally upon two specific cell types: B cells and T cells that respond to specific antigens. The adaptive immune system is involved in turning off the inflammatory response with anti-inflammatory cytokines and chemokines. This allows for phase changes; for example, in innate immune cells such as macrophages, where in the innate environment they are polarized in an M1 phase (proinflammatory phenotype) with poor phagocytosis. In the adaptive phase, macrophages are in the M2 phase (anti-inflammatory phenotype) and are primed with phagocytosis cleaning up the cellular debris and removing viruses and bacteria with attached antibodies. Again, whereas the innate system response, including inflammation and the release of cytokines, occurs within minutes or hours of contact with a pathogen, the adaptive immune responses occur after several days, when they are triggered to take over or help the innate system. In general, the adaptive response entails several discrete steps, including

1. recognition of the antigen,

2. release of white blood cells (lymphocytes; the most significant TReg differentiation),

3. activation and proliferation of responding cells,

4. gene transcription,

5. synthesis of proteins, and

6. production of specific end products, such as antibodies and cytokines.

Further, since immune cells need to migrate to specific locations within the body in response to infection or injury, the process of chemotaxis relies on redox balance to help immune cells move toward a site of inflammation or infection, ensuring an effective immune response. As we've seen, redox balance plays an important role in controlling inflammation. While an appropriate inflammatory response is necessary for defense against pathogens, excessive and prolonged inflammation can be harmful. Redox signaling helps modulate inflammatory pathways, contributing to the resolution of inflammation once the threat is eliminated. ROS generated by immune cells such as macrophages serve as part of the immune response against pathogens. Redox balance is essential to ensure the controlled production of ROS, preventing excessive damage to host tissues. Redox balance influences the activation and function of cells in the adaptive immune system, including T cells and B cells. Proper redox regulation is crucial for the development of an effective and specific immune response.

## THE IMPORTANCE OF SLEEP FOR REDOX BALANCE

While we may all agree that sleep is important to our overall health, what sleep does for the brain and body is complex; indeed, sleep researchers have not yet come to clear consensus on the biological roots of sleep or how best to address and support the intricacies of its process. And though we know that the quality and duration of sleep matter, there is much more to understand about its functions to truly appreciate how sleep affects almost every system in the body.

### The Sleep Drive

In "Sleep Drive Is Encoded by Neural Plastic Changes in a Dedicated Circuit," Wu and colleagues at Johns Hopkins use the concept of homeostasis to frame a comprehensive understanding of how and why the sleep drive is so important to overall health and how it intersects with the circadian clock to either promote high-quality sleep or undermine it. As they point out, "The nature of the sleep drive itself remains unclear . . . unraveling the processes encoding the sleep drive requires an understanding of both how the sleep drive is generated and how it persists."

So what is the sleep drive? It's our natural desire and need for sleep, which is related to the probability or likelihood of falling asleep when we go to bed. Typically, the odds of falling asleep are predicted or measured by the gradual accumulation of a specific neurotransmitter, adenosine, a nucleoside, which is one of four building blocks of RNA and is generated in the cystol of neurons as a by-product of metabolic exhaustion. In short, when we are physically and mentally tired our cells are depleted of energy, and adenosine triggers the need and desire to go to sleep. At a cellular level, adenosine relaxes and dilates the blood vessels and slows the heartbeat and generates anti-inflammatory activity. The breakdown of ATP in the brain produces the metabolite adenosine. Adenosine then activates A1 and A2A receptors in the nucleus accumbens and hypothalmus of the brain, inhibiting arousal and neural activity and enhancing slow-wave deep sleep.

The sleep drive is expressed as an accumulation of pressure that builds up throughout the day and only dissipates during sleep. It is thought to be regulated by a complex network of molecular pathways and physiological processes that involve both the circadian clock and homeostatic mechanisms. Experts such as Wu and colleagues identified a specific neural circuit in the brain that is involved in regulating the sleep drive. This circuit involves the neurotransmitter dopamine, which is known to play a role in regulating reward and motivation, as well as in promoting wakefulness. In one study, the researchers used optogenetics, a technique that allows for the precise control of neural activity using light, to manipulate the activity of dopamine neurons in mice and examine the effects on sleep behavior. They found that increasing the activity of dopamine neurons during wakefulness led to an increase in the sleep drive, while decreasing the activity of dopamine neurons during wakefulness led to a decrease in the sleep drive.

Furthermore, the researchers found that the plasticity of this circuit is critical for encoding the sleep drive. They showed that sleep deprivation led to an increase in the density of synapses, the connections between neurons, in this circuit, which in turn increased the sensitivity of dopamine neurons to sleep pressure. This plasticity is thought to be a critical mechanism for adapting to changes in sleep patterns and maintaining the balance between sleep and wakefulness.

Gamma-aminobutyric acid (GABA) and histamine are two additional neurotransmitters that play an important role in sleep regulation. GABA promotes sleep by inhibiting wake-promoting neurons and is thought to be involved in the regulation of the sleep drive. Histamine promotes wakefulness by activating wake-promoting neurons. The release of histamine is inhibited during sleep and increases during wakefulness, thus contributing to the sleep–wake cycle and the regulation of the sleep drive.

Overall, the regulation of the sleep drive is complex and involves many different neurotransmitters and other molecular pathways. Adenosine, GABA, dopamine, and histamine are just a few examples of the many neurotransmitters that play a role in this process. However, importantly, the modulation of these neurotransmitters depends to a large degree on redox homeostasis and points to the importance of another feature of sleep, the circadian clock.

## The Centrality of the Circadian Clock

As physicians and healthcare providers, we know that people who regularly work at night and sleep during the day suffer from more illnesses and diseases than their day-shift counterparts. In our practices, we also are seeing more and more patients with metabolic syndrome, diabetes, and heart and blood pressure issues. And while these conditions can have genetic etiologies, they often are directly related to lifestyle behaviors such as smoking, lack of regular exercise, poor diet, and poor sleep hygiene. For people who alternate between day shift and night shift, these conditions are exacerbated. In fact, what's becoming clearer in recent studies is that the cluster of these conditions can actually be traced to circadian clock disruption.

In short, the circadian clock mechanism—both its central clock in the suprachiasmatic nucleus (SCN) of the hypothalamus and the peripheral clocks in cells distributed throughout the body—controls a number of elemental biological processes, including the sleep–wake cycle, body temperature, hormone secretion and functioning, digestion, metabolic homeostasis (especially tied to glucose metabolism), and proper immune functioning. When any aspect of the circadian clock becomes disrupted—by working nights, for example—a domino effect of negative reactions can occur at the cellular level.

It's worth noting that more than 15% of Americans rely on shift work, which points to the pervasiveness of this problem. As our systems try to stay in homeostatic balance, the regulatory mechanisms that drive cell functioning become "misaligned," with serious consequences for cells, tissues, and whole-organism function. At the cellular level, cell functioning is impacted and has been directly tied to conditions such as metabolic syndrome, diabetes, cardiovascular disease, cancer, and intestinal disorders. As the authors of a recent paper point out, "The increased prevalence of diseases associated with circadian disruption underscores the need to better understand how circadian disruption can wreak havoc in so many different ways throughout the body." The balance of redox has a profound effect on the circadian clock; clock genes turn on ATP production in the morning and NADPH production at night.

## How Sleep Dysregulation Affects Cell Functioning

What happens when the circadian clock gets disrupted? First, the body works harder to stay regulated, interrupting the normal catabolic and anabolic processes of basic energy metabolism. As a result, maintaining a balance of cellular redox becomes more challenging. Down the line, this exertion or use of cellular energy taxes redox, depletes enzymatic chains, and ultimately impacts the immune response. The combination of inefficient glucose metabolism and high blood pressure wears on at least two basic systems that affect both heart health and digestive/brain health. And further down the line, epigenetic changes can begin to appear.

At the cellular level, the mechanisms of the circadian clock are auto-regulated and tied to cyclic expressions of so-called "clock genes," which together make up the molecular clock. Over a 24-hour period, proteins are called to stimulate and repress production. These clock-controlled genes help to regulate lipid and cholesterol biosynthesis, carbohydrate metabolism, oxidative phosphorylation, and glucose levels—all related to maintaining redox balance.

Also keep in mind that circadian rhythms are widely distributed and affect many systems peripherally, including adipose tissue, the pancreas, the liver, the heart, and parts of the immune system.

The potential danger of disruption of peripheral circadian clocks is great because they directly regulate up to 20% of the genome. In addition, the clock network is integrated within all of the major cellular signaling and metabolic pathways (see Table 1).

**Table 1.** Molecules Impacting Wakefulness and Sleep

| WAKEFULNESS | SLEEP |
|---|---|
| Acetylcholine | Proinflammatory cytokines |
| Norepinephrine | GABA |
| Hypocretins | Prostaglandins |
| Glutamate | Adenosine |
| | Extracellular ATP |
| | Nitrous oxide (NO) |

## A Cellular Deep Dive into Circadian Disruption

In addition to metabolic, heart, and immune conditions that are either triggered or exacerbated by circadian disruption, several other concerning comorbidities can occur.

*Alcohol-Induced Circadian Disruption*

Conditions such as liver disease caused by alcohol consumption can often be traced back to alcohol-induced circadian disruption, caused by mechanisms necessary to metabolize alcohol and the consequent negative adaptations in the intestinal lining. Although alcohol metabolism takes place mostly in the liver, the stomach, intestine, and brain are also involved in this process at a cellular level.

For instance, alcohol metabolism will cause a shift in the cellular ratio of NAD+ to NADH because of how SIRT1 is highly sensitive to the cellular ratio of NAD+ to NADH. In other words, NAD+ levels will decrease as a result of alcohol metabolism by alcohol dehyd (LADH) and aldeheyde dehydrogense (ADH). People who drink put a big burden on the NAD/NADPH ratio because of the pull from the NAD pool. Further, alcohol downgrades the intestinal lining, causing intestinal hyperpermeability, which then permits luminal bacterial contents such as endotoxins (e.g., lipopolysaccharide) to translocate through the intestinal epithelium into the systemic circulation. These endotoxins further disrupt circadian rhythms.

### Downgrading of Immunity

A disruption of circadian rhythms also undermines immune function. In general, irregular sleep–wake cycles alter the normal circadian rhythmicity of immune cells and increase the susceptibility to infections. In studies, chronically shifting light–dark cycles in mice augmented lipopolysaccharide-induced immune response, resulting in greater mortality compared with non-circadian-disrupted mice.

### Overweight and Obesity

Eating at night or continually throughout the day can upset the circadian rhythmicity and disrupt the clock, and has been linked to weight gain, obesity, and metabolic syndrome. In studies, mice fed during an inappropriate time gained more weight than mice fed during an appropriate time, despite similar activity levels and caloric intake. This phenomenon is also observed in humans; people who skip breakfast and have eating patterns shifted toward late-night eating tend to be more overweight than those who consume food during more appropriate time periods.

### Epigenetic Changes

As mentioned above, shift work can instigate a host of downstream effects on cell functioning and cause disorders. One of these downstream effects can be epigenetic in origin and trigger tumor growth. Epigenetic changes also occur as a consequence of chronic circadian disruption in the promoter regions of genes encoding glucocorticoid receptors (important for hypothalamic–pituitary–adrenal axis function), TNFalpha (a cytokine critical for cell functioning and inflammation), and IFNgamma. Changes such as these may play a critical role in how chronic circadian disruption promotes cancer, inflammation, and metabolic disorders.

Circadian clock disruption can create epigenetic changes to cellular pathways, which in turn impact overall functioning and efficiency. When cells are forced to compromise to maintain homeostasis, intervening with peptides, for example, can positively affect redox balance and overall homeostatic health of the cells and their pathways. Remember, the epigenome is distinct from the genome. We do have the power to interrupt negative epigenetic changes; it's the genome whose changes are not reversible.

This lens of epigenetics offers us a way to intervene before damage to the genome occurs and disease develops. Indeed, the shift worker is like a living laboratory, embodying many conditions and opportunities for rectification.

## Sleep Apnea

Sleep disturbance can be caused by a variety of factors, such as stress and anxiety, poor sleep habits, medical conditions, medications, and sleep disorders. While sleep apnea is a relatively common cause of sleep disturbance, it is important to note that not all sleep disturbance is caused by sleep apnea. Other sleep disorders, such as insomnia and restless leg syndrome, as well as medical conditions such as chronic pain and gastroesophageal reflux disease (GERD), can also contribute to sleep disturbance. However, sleep apnea is a prevalent presentation of poor sleep with common symptoms such as snoring, gasping or choking during sleep, and excessive daytime sleepiness.

The most common cause of sleep apnea is obstructive sleep apnea (OSA), which occurs when the airway becomes partially or completely blocked during sleep, leading to breathing pauses and disrupted sleep. The blockage is often caused by relaxation and collapse of the tongue and soft tissues in the back of the throat, which can narrow or completely obstruct the airway.

Risk factors for OSA include obesity, older age, male gender, family history of sleep apnea, smoking, alcohol and sedative use, and certain anatomical features such as a narrow airway or large tonsils. Less commonly, sleep apnea can be caused by central sleep apnea (CSA), which occurs when the brain fails to send signals to the muscles responsible for breathing. CSA is often associated with underlying medical conditions such as heart failure or neurological disorders.

Mouth breathing during sleep can cause the tongue and soft tissues in the back of the throat to relax and collapse, leading to airway obstruction and snoring. Additionally, mouth breathing can cause the tissues in the upper airway to become dry and inflamed, which can further narrow the airway and exacerbate sleep apnea.

It is difficult to determine the exact percentage of sleep apnea patients who are primarily mouth breathers, as this can vary depending on the individual and the underlying cause of their sleep apnea. However, it is generally believed that mouth breathing can contribute to the development or worsening of sleep apnea in some individuals.

Some studies have suggested that mouth breathing may be more common in individuals with certain types of sleep apnea, such as positional obstructive sleep apnea (POSA). POSA occurs when the airway becomes partially or completely blocked when an individual sleeps in a certain position and is often associated with mouth breathing.

Sleep apnea is a serious condition that can cause disrupted sleep and lead to a host of health issues if left untreated. While treatments such as CPAP machines and dental devices can be effective, they can also be difficult to use and costly. However, recent research has suggested that a simple solution may be available in the form of mouth taping. Mouth taping involves placing tape over the mouth before sleep, which can help to promote nasal breathing and reduce the likelihood of airway obstruction. When individuals breathe through their mouth during sleep, the tongue and soft tissues in the back of the throat may relax and block the airway, leading to snoring and sleep apnea. By encouraging nasal breathing, mouth taping may help to keep the airway open and reduce the frequency and severity of breathing pauses during sleep. Additionally, mouth taping may help to improve the alignment of the jaw and tongue, further reducing the likelihood of airway obstruction. While more research is needed to fully understand the safety and effectiveness of mouth taping, it may offer a simple and cost-effective solution for some individuals with OSA.

Recent studies and a review article provide evidence to support the use of mouth taping as a therapy for OSA. In a 2021 study published in the *Journal of Clinical Sleep Medicine*, 72 individuals with mild to moderate OSA were randomly assigned to either a mouth-taping group or a control group. The mouth-taping group had significantly reduced Apnea-Hypopnea Index (AHI) scores and improved oxygen saturation levels compared to the control group, suggesting that mouth taping may be a low-cost and noninvasive therapy for mild to moderate OSA. A 2020 review article in the same journal noted that mouth taping may be a viable option for individuals who are unable or unwilling to use other therapies such as CPAP, particularly for mouth breathers. However, the authors caution that mouth taping should only be undertaken under the guidance of a healthcare professional and should be carefully monitored for safety and efficacy. A 2019 article in the *Journal of Dental Sleep Medicine* discussed the use of mouth taping as a therapy for snoring and sleep apnea, noting that it may be effective in reducing snoring and promoting nasal breathing but may not be effective for all individuals with sleep apnea.

## THE BENEFITS OF SUPPORTING REDOX BALANCE

In the pages ahead, I will show how 30 powerful supplements can support energy metabolism, cellular redox, microbiome balance, and immune modulation. You will also discover how eating an alkaline-balanced diet; intermittent fasting; specific, well-timed exercise; and proper sleep hygiene can further support redox pathways. Together, these components make up The Redox Promise, whose goal is to

- fight cancer,
- improve the modulation and balance of the innate and adaptive immune systems,
- sustain our attention and focus,
- increase mental and physical energy,
- sharpen our memory,

- improve the quality of our sleep,

- help us lose weight,

- strengthen our bones, muscles, and joints,

- grow our hair and nails,

- rejuvenate our skin, and

- ease pain.

As much as everyone would love to hear that there is a magic pill or one activity or one special food that will do it all when it comes to cellular health and vitality, I am here to say that there isn't and to run away when this is pitched. On the other hand, adding a few supplements at the right time in rotation, getting good nutrition, exercising regularly, and getting sufficient deep sleep will move the needle on our health. We will feel immediate results: more energy, clearer focus, improved well-being, and a baseline for better aging.

Healthy aging requires a commitment to our own self-care. It also takes discipline, but with that discipline can come tremendous rewards. As you learn about some familiar and unfamiliar supplements, it's important to advise your patients to start by introducing a few at a time and rotating small groups of them. Then, read on to find out how the integration of resistance strength training and aerobic exercise, a healthy diet, fasting, sufficient sleep, and stress reduction work synergistically to protect us from environmental assaults and help us achieve the cellular wellness of optimal efficiency, flexibility, and protection.

# 30 Supplements That **Optimize Health** and **Regenerate** the Brain and Body



## PART 2

The 30 supplements covered here support the cellular health of the brain and body and enable better aging. Each works on a specific attribute of cell functioning—enhancing cell efficiency, targeting cell dysfunction, and supporting cellular redox balance.

Most of these supplements are compounds that our brain or body produces naturally when given proper, well-rounded nutrition; however, as we age, the cells of the body stop producing these compounds or don't produce them in effective amounts. This is the simple reason for supplementation: giving the body what we know it needs. Most of the supplements are in the form of a tablet or powder, and nearly all are easily obtained at specialty pharmacies or through online retailers and do not require a prescription. The only exception is lactulose, which requires a prescription. I do recommend checking labels and sources of the product ingredients, and choosing high-quality, reputable producers known for their ethics and purity of ingredients. And always follow the recommended dosage stipulated on the label.

It's important that as a trusted medical provider, you educate yourself on the nuances of each of the supplements and be guided by how best to address your patients' issues or challenges with maintaining cellular redox. I can't emphasize enough the importance of rotating groups of supplements. In the dosage instructions, you will note which supplements should be taken in rotation. Often, patients come to me taking a kitchen sink approach to supplements, as if more is better. In response, I often tell these patients to take fewer supplements and instead focus on timing and rotation of key supplements, so they don't interfere with redox balance. Trust both the subjective and objective data from your patients when assessing supplementation benefits.

When beginning a new supplement, patients should take the time to read about how it works and what it targets. I recommend that you have your patients choose one or two at a time, depending on their needs, and that they give themselves a week or two to see how they feel. It's also wise to make sure your patients include additional members of their healthcare team when adding or changing their regimen, especially if they take medicines regularly for various conditions. I also encourage you to share this book with other practitioners so that they can learn about the importance of redox, the supplements and their pathways, and the positive health outcomes they can provide. Many patients when they first come to see me present in an over-reduced state from self-prescribing too many antioxidants.

## 1-MNA

A variant of vitamin B3, 1-methylnicotinamide (1-MNA) is produced by the body when the body shifts from carbohydrate metabolism into fat metabolism, as happens as a consequence of calorie restriction or exercise. 1-MNA's role in metabolism can be understood within the context of how the body manages energy.

In the field of metabolic science, a significant study has shed light on the relationship between diet, exercise, and energy management in the body. 1-MNA is the by-product of a substance called nicotinamide N-methyltransferase (NNMT). The focus of this research was on the role of NNMT and 1-MNA in the relationship between diet, exercise, and energy management. The study revealed that when we restrict calorie intake and engage in activity, there is an increase in NNMT expression in our muscles, which leads to higher levels of 1-MNA. This discovery emphasizes the role of NNMT—and therefore the role of 1-MNA—in how the body adapts to varying energy demands.

1-MNA also helps regulate glucose levels. In studies involving diabetes patients, researchers have found that 1-MNA has the potential to lower fasting glucose levels, suggesting it could be used as a treatment for managing diabetes; indeed, one study proposes that 1-MNA could be a biomarker for assessing metabolic flexibility and detecting metabolic diseases at an early stage, as it is correlated with both body mass index and insulin sensitivity.

Research has also shown the benefits of using 1-MNA for treating kidney damage in cases where there is ongoing protein loss in urine, a condition known as *refractory proteinuria*. In addition, 1-MNA has been associated with a reduction in oxidative stress, cell death, and inflammation. Research has also highlighted the protective role of 1-MNA: In heart cells experiencing oxidative stress and inflammation, 1-MNA was effective in mitigating the harmful effects of a high-fat diet.

Furthermore, the formation of 1-MNA triggered by muscle activity in mice highlights its significance in relation to exercise and physical exertion. Based on these discoveries, scientists think that incorporating 1-MNA supplements could potentially protect against illness; indeed, studies show that 1-MNA has improved recovery after intense exercise as well as viruses such as COVID-19. Essentially, by supplementing with 1 MNA, the body can produce more NAD via the salvage pathway; this will make NAD+ more available when needed in the cell. At the same time, the methylation pool will be improved and more methylation will be available when needed. Lastly, 1 MNA has a metabolic role and directly activates SIRT 1 and SIRT 3 proteins for deacteylation, which is so important for ATP and NAD+ reduction in redox. (SIRT 1 and SIRT 3 are NAD+ dependent.)

## Dosage

In terms of commercial 1-MNA supplements, the Polish supplement brand Endothelia offers a 58-mg dosage of 1-MNA per capsule. It's important to note that the optimal dosage of 1-MNA as a supplement hasn't been fully established, and more research is needed to determine the most effective and safest dosages. However, it's worth mentioning that Endothelia's supplement received approval from the European Commission in 2018 to introduce 1-MNA as an ingredient in novel foods in the European Union. This approval indicates that the supplement meets the safety and quality standards required for sale and consumption in Europe.

## ACETYL L-CARNITINE

Acetyl L-carnitine, also known as ALCAR, is a derivative of an amino acid that plays a role in how the body generates energy, enhances memory, and uplifts mood. Acetyl L-carnitine has been shown to offset cognitive impairment and the symptoms of Alzheimer's disease.

Research has also shown that acetyl L-carnitine has the potential to protect the brain–body system from the dangers of neurotoxicity, oxidative stress, and chronic inflammation. Studies have shown that acetyl L-carnitine increases insulin sensitivity, which in turn may reverse type 2 diabetes and improve heart health. The effectiveness of acetyl L-carnitine in improving function may be attributed to its ability to cross the blood–brain barrier and enhance the production of neurotransmitters such as acetylcholine and dopamine, therefore helping to reduce pain.

Acetyl L-carnitine also improves oxidation of fat utilization by the mitochondria to make cells more efficient at cell signaling and acts as a mitochondrial antioxidant, improving cellular redox. ALCAR also helps in membrane stabilization and contributes to glycogen replenishment, helping speed recovery. In addition, acetyl L-carnitine has been used to boost exercise performance through increased energy production while reducing muscle damage and post-workout fatigue. And for those on a weight loss journey, acetyl L-carnitine can be a trusted companion by boosting metabolism and aiding in fat burning while replenishing glycogen.

## Dosage

While individual requirements may vary depending on health status and specific goals, there are some guidelines supported by research. For promoting brain functions, daily doses ranging from 1.5 to 4.5 g have shown results. To alleviate pain, a daily dosage of 1 to 3 g has been shown to be effective. When it comes to weight loss and athletic performance enhancement, recommended doses usually range from 2 to 3 g and from 1.5 to 3 g, respectively. Acetyl L-carnitine comes in capsule and powder forms. This supplement is best used in a cycle of 3 months on, 6 weeks off. I use ARCAL rather than L-carnitine; the research supports better brain penetration with ALCAR.

# AKG

Alpha ketoglutarate (AKG) isn't just any old molecule. This powerful supplement has the ability to heal wounds more quickly, strengthen the body's immune defenses, sharpen mental abilities, fight against osteoporosis, maintain muscle mass, resist sarcopenia, and improve athletic performance. Importantly, AKG also supports the female reproductive system. As something the body already produces, it plays a crucial role in the complex web of metabolic processes taking place in our body.

When it comes to the process of wound healing, AKG steps in by promoting collagen synthesis, which is essential for proper healing. It can also reduce inflammation and oxidative stress, two factors that can slow down healing. AKG also plays a role in maintaining proper redox balance. By activating the NRF2 pathway and removing molecules, promoting antioxidant production, and enhancing function, AKG acts as a protector of cellular integrity.

Our immune system acts as a shield against threats, and AKG might be just what it needs to stay strong. Studies have shown that it can effectively regulate the activity of cells such as T cells and macrophages—key players in defending the body against infections and diseases. In this way, AKG holds promising anticancer effects presently being studied. Furthermore, it may help to combat brain fog by increasing the production of neurotransmitters such as dopamine and serotonin.

AKG also is known to combat stress, further positioning it as an agent for better aging. Because of its help in modulating DNA repair pathways and the expression of genes, it can also be antitumor. In fact, in the fight against cancer progression, AKG demonstrates its impact by regulating a transcription factor called hypoxia factor (HIF). AKG feeds directly into the Krebs cycle, which is vital to ATP production. HIF plays a role in metabolism, angiogenesis (the formation of new blood vessels), and cell survival. Normally, HIF is targeted at elimination. With low oxygen conditions or the presence of AKG, this elimination process is halted. As a result, HIF becomes stabilized and activated, thereby leading to increased gene transcription that's crucial for angiogenesis, glycolysis (glucose metabolism), and cell survival.

I also recommend AKG for the elite-level athletes I work with. By boosting energy production and reducing muscle breakdown, it not only enhances performance but also eases muscle soreness and fatigue for quicker recovery.

## Dosage

While specific dosages may vary depending on the purpose, studies have provided some recommendations. To support better aging and enhance cell function, the suggested daily dosages are 3 to 6 g. For performance, a daily intake of 6 to 20 g appears beneficial. AKG plays a role in bone density and preventing osteoporosis at a dosage of 6 to 12 g daily. Further research will continue to finesse these recommendations. There are two types of AKG: calcium and arginine. My preference is to use arginine in supplementation because it enhances nitric oxide production, which is an important cell signaling agent for maintaining collagen, bone stimulation, muscle formation, and immune modulation.

## AMINO DRINK

While drinking eight glasses of water each day is helpful for keeping our metabolism running smoothly and maintaining energy levels, there's more to hydration than quenching our thirst. Enter the Amino Drink, a blend of fluids, electrolytes, and amino acids that is a powerful better-aging agent.

This power drink offers a refreshing hint of lemon and is designed to give the body and mind an extra boost. My top-notch athletes swear by its properties, noting how it aids in recovery after intense workouts; similarly, my orthopedic patients find comfort in its healing abilities. And as our lives remain overshadowed by COVID-19 and other nasty viruses, the Amino Drink acts as a shield by preparing the liver to combat infections and reducing the duration of illnesses. Cellular hydration (swelling) decreases a virus's ability to penetrate and replicate.

Let's take a look at the science behind the Amino Drink and delve into *cell osmolarity*, a term that refers to cell swelling that accompanies adequate hydration. When cells expand due to proper fluid intake, they not only help cleanse the system but also cause the cell membrane to become hyperpolarized, which enhances optimal communication between cells. This improved communication aids in the rejuvenation of liver cells. It's important to remember that the liver works tirelessly to detoxify the body, and like any hardworking entity, it occasionally requires support. When liver cells, called *hepatocytes*, swell they become more efficient at detoxifying the body. Imagine the capability of every cell having this opportunity to increase its efficiency with swelling—including its amazing influence on the muscle cells (myocytes).

Numerous studies emphasize the importance of cell swelling and how it enhances health and cellular functionality. When cells expand due to increased hydration, they are better able to utilize amino acids, which in turn equips cells with nutrients to maintain their activity and vibrancy.

Specifically, as hepatocytes swell, they initiate signals that increase the production of certain enzymes crucial for detoxification, such as cytochrome P450s. An increased presence of these enzymes enables the liver to neutralize toxins better. Moreover, this swelling makes the cell membrane more flexible and assists proteins and receptors on the cell surface in functioning more effectively. This is essential for eliminating substances from the body—a crucial feature of maintaining redox balance and overall cellular homeostasis, both key to better aging.

Interestingly, hepatocytes have a mechanism for maintaining their size. If they swell excessively, they release some water and other solutes that can aid in eliminating waste products. Another advantage of this swelling is that it promotes the flow of bile, a liquid that plays a role in eliminating toxins. The microbiome metabolizes bile into secondary metabolites that are important in maintaining cellular redox (see the upcoming section "TUDCA" for more on this topic). This process also increases the energy production of cells, providing them with the power to facilitate detoxification reactions that require energy. Additionally, this process triggers defense mechanisms within cells, resulting in increased levels of antioxidants and protective proteins. These mechanisms ensure that cells remain healthy and efficient while detoxifying. Drinking the Amino Drink two or three times per week can make a positive difference in your cell metabolism. Again, most of the science validates cellular swelling in hepatocytes improving liver function; the science also supports muscle cell swelling (optimal hydration of myocytes) improving muscle function and adaption, which in turn improves performance and recovery.

## Dosage

Here's a step-by-step guide to preparing this elixir:

1. Begin by selecting a 48-ounce or half gallon (1.5 liter) jug, a water bottle, or any large container filled with purified water.

2. Add the following amino acids to the container:

- 4 g L-glycine
- 3 g L-glutamine (some athletes gradually increase this to 10 to 15 g over the course of a few weeks for improved performance and rehabilitation)
- 5 g L-alanine
- 5 g creatine (a combination of methionine, arginine, and glycine)
- 3 g L-leucine

3. For electrolyte replenishment, add ¼ cup of coconut water to the mixture for a boost without any added sugars. You can also use an electrolyte packet that contains no added sugars.

4. Finish by adding a squeeze of lemon juice for some tang and/or 1 tsp trehalose for taste. (Trehalose improves hydration of the cell.)

I prepare a batch of Amino Drink every morning and enjoy it throughout the day. However, please note that it is best to avoid storing this mixture in the refrigerator for more than 1 day as the amino acids may degrade over time. Embrace this health elixir and unlock the secret to improved well-being!

## BICARBONATE

Bicarbonate, aka hydrogen carbonate, is a chemical compound that offers multiple health advantages. First, bicarbonate in the form of Alka Seltzer Gold or baking soda, providing relief to individuals suffering from reflux and heartburn. (However, Alka-Selzter Gold is better on the stomach; baking soda can cause stomach upset.)

Second, bicarbonate plays a role in redox reactions. Because bicarbonate helps regulate pH levels, it supports the antioxidant system and enhances the functioning of mitochondria, which are vital for generating energy and protect against the high acid content of the typical Western diet. Meats, dairy, sugar, and other simple carbohydrates increase the acid load within the gut, which negatively affects muscle tissues and bones. However, bicarbonate steps in as a buffer against this acid, safeguarding both muscle tissue and bone health.

The incredible properties of bicarbonate also help to maintain the body's pH balance, ensuring that the blood stays at a healthy pH level. This is essential for the functioning of our organs, especially the kidneys, which act as the body's natural filtration system. By preventing the formation of kidney stones and reducing the risk of kidney diseases, bicarbonate acts as a guardian for kidney health. Athletes can also take advantage of its benefits, because research has shown that it alleviates muscle fatigue and enhances endurance.

Bicarbonate also promotes dental and skin health. Its gentle abrasive nature makes it highly effective in removing surface stains from teeth, thereby promoting health. Additionally, its exfoliating properties ensure that the skin remains revitalized and free from the burden of dead skin cells.

## Dosage

Determining the dosage of bicarbonate depends on several factors, including a person's specific health condition, age, weight, and overall well-being. Typically, the recommended daily intake is 500 to 1000 mg of bicarbonate spread out over three meals. However, it's important to note that excessive consumption can lead to side effects such as diarrhea. The idea is to consume enough to balance your gut.

If taking bicarbonate to help improve performance during intense exercise, the suggested dose usually falls within the range of 0.2 to 0.4 g per kg of body weight. I recommend taking it 1 hour before exercising.

If taking bicarbonate in the form of Alka Seltzer Gold, the recommended dose is 2 tablets every 4 hours as needed, up to three times daily. Do not exceed 6 tablets in 24 hours.

While baking soda can also be used as a form of bicarbonate, its dosage should be closely monitored to prevent discomfort. Microdosing with baking soda has been shown to enhance athletic performance, with fewer side effects—but this takes great preparation and execution. With time and regular use, however, individuals can adapt without experiencing any distress.

## BOVINE COLOSTRUM

The benefits of bovine colostrum stem from research on human colostrum, the substance produced by the mammary glands and secreted to infants while nursing. Human colostrum is known to contain a wealth of immune-supporting ingredients that mothers can give to their infants in the hours, days, and months after birth.

Bovine colostrum shares some of these immune-supporting properties, especially as it strengthens the gut lining and prevents permeability. This can lead to improved absorption and overall improved gut function, which is especially important for individuals with compromised gut integrity. One standout ingredient of bovine colostrum is lactoferrin, a glycoprotein that binds to iron and offers an antimicrobial effect, supporting the growth of beneficial gut bacteria. Lactoferrin also plays a role in gut health by influencing cytokine and chemokine levels through its properties and interactions with immune cells. Specifically, bovine colostrum provides immunoglobulins, lactoferrin, lysozyme, lactoperoxidase, microRNA glycoconjugates, B and T lymphocytes, leukocytes, interleukins, and other valuable polypeptides. The growth factors present in colostrum stimulate cell growth, proliferation, healing processes, and cell differentiation, as well as provide an essential source of macronutrients including proteins, fats, and carbohydrates along with some vitamins and minerals.

Bovine colostrum also contains omega-3 and omega-6 fatty acids and short-chain fatty acids (SCFAs), adding to its nutritional benefits.

Bovine colostrum can also be used topically. It contains components such as nucleotides, epidermal growth factor (EGF), transforming growth factor (TGF), and insulin-like growth factor 1 (IGF-1), which promote cellular and skin growth while aiding in DNA and RNA repair. Overall, bovine colostrum serves as an ally when it comes to fortifying our system. Various studies have shown that bovine colostrum is effective in reducing the risk of respiratory infections in both children and adults. This suggests that it has potential as a therapeutic agent for immune-related conditions.

Bovine colostrum proves to be a substance with a range of health benefits. Its impact on gut permeability, its inflammatory properties, and its potential for enhancing athletic performance and overall well-being are just the beginning.

## Dosage

I recommend a dosage of 1 packet (2 g) daily to start, and then working up to 6 g daily. Patients will see and feel an improvement in their skin, sleep, digestion, and hair and nail growth. Another source of bovine colostrum is colostrum liposomal delivery powder (5g dosage). Since this is a food group and therefore a source of nutrition, it can be taken indefinitely.

## BUTYRATE

Within the field of medicine lies a compound with the potential to revolutionize our understanding of well-being and overall health. This compound is butyrate, a short-chain fatty acid (SCFA) that offers us an agent for healthy aging on multiple fronts.

Produced in the colon, butyrate is considered a post-biotic, derived through the fermentation of fiber by certain types of bacteria that live in the gut. Research has shown that certain fibers, such as starch, which evades digestion in the intestine and is fermented by gut bacteria, have particularly strong effects on boosting butyrate levels. Similarly effective is inulin, a fructooligosaccharide (FOS), which is a type of fructan that undergoes fermentation in the intestine. Pectin, found in fruits and vegetables, along with beta-glucans, found in grains such as oats and barley, have also been proven to be promoters of butyrate production.

Why do I place importance on butyrate? At its core, butyrate provides energy to the cells that line the colon and serves as a foundation for maintaining healthy gut microbiota. It also possesses a remarkable ability to combat inflammation and oxidative stress by promoting the development of T cells and therefore supporting the immune response. Ingesting butyrate will help defend against conditions such as inflammatory bowel disease (IBD) and leaky gut syndrome and ensures healthy bowel movements.

Butyrate also has significant anti-inflammatory properties and promotes redox processes within cells. Its activation of the NRF2 pathway, inhibition of the NF-κB pathway, impact on histone acetylation regulation, and influence on gut bacteria reflect its approach to maintaining health, helping to regulate genes, and modulating cytokine production. By reducing levels of inflammatory cytokines such as TNFalpha and IL-6 while increasing anti-inflammatory agents such as IL10 and TGF-beta, butyrate helps maintain a delicate balance in the body's inflammatory response. Furthermore, its ability to inhibit histone deacetylase (HDAC) leads to changes in histone acetylation that activate genes associated with reducing inflammation. This gives hope to individuals battling conditions such as Crohn's disease and ulcerative colitis.

Butyrate can also be an aid to weight loss, as it helps to regulate hormones that affect appetite and fat storage. By increasing the production of gut hormones such as peptide YY (PYY) and glucagon-like peptide-1 (GLP-1), which help control appetite, it creates a feeling of fullness and may reduce calorie intake. Additionally, its interaction with the AMP-activated protein kinase (AMPK) enzyme aids in increased burning and decreased storage of fats.

New research suggests that butyrate may improve mood and lessen symptoms of depression and anxiety. Its influence on the connection between the gut and brain (known as the gut–brain axis), regulation of factors such as brain-derived neurotrophic factor (BDNF), and anti-inflammatory actions highlight its potential role as a therapeutic agent for emotion regulation.

Butyrate activates the mTOR pathway and stimulates the secretion of growth hormone, preventing muscle breakdown and enhancing muscle mass and strength. This makes it a valuable ally for athletes and those who exercise regularly. And given its anti-inflammatory properties, butyrate can improve performance and speed up recovery.

Recent research also suggests that butyrate has the potential to fight colorectal cancer by inhibiting the growth of colon cancer cells through inducing cell death, blocking cell multiplication, and suppressing blood vessel formation. Additionally, its influence on gut bacteria balance and its ability to inhibit HDAC enzymes make it a formidable opponent of this type of cancer.

## Dosage

My general recommendation for all my patients is to start with 1.2 g per meal and not to exceed 9 g daily (there is a liquid form, but it is harder to access). Dosing is dependent on the patient's microbiome health. If someone does not show signs of dysbiosis, they are probably producing butyrate sufficiently, though you can perform a DNA test for butyrate production. (When testing, look for DNA of whole genome sequencing instead of RNA sequencing, to ensure better accuracy.)

When addressing bowel disease (e.g., IBD), typical recommendations for oral supplementation range from 2 to 4 g daily of sodium butyrate divided into two or three doses. It's important to note that actual dosages may vary depending on symptom severity and individual patient response.

Cancer prevention clinical trials have utilized doses ranging from 3 to 4 g daily using forms such as tributyrin or sodium butyrate. In terms of metabolic disorders, daily sodium butyrate intake usually falls within the range of 2 to 4 g.

## COLLAGEN PEPTIDES

Collagen peptides are all the rage, but it's important to understand how these remarkable compounds support our overall health and healthy aging. Collagen peptides help maintain skin elasticity, ensuring hydration and improving overall skin texture. Moreover, collagen is a component of cartilage, which is vital for joint health; indeed, research has shown that regular consumption of collagen peptides reduces pain and stiffness and protects against conditions such as osteoarthritis. I often hear from patients that other doctors have said that ingestion of collagen hydroxylate has no health benefits; this is easily refuted by the well-documented literature.

Collagen peptides also show promise in promoting bone health. Since collagen helps build bones, supplementation can strengthen bone density and decrease the risk of fractures, particularly among postmenopausal females. Studies indicate that supplementing with collagen peptides can also enhance muscle mass and strength. Collagen peptides contain important amino acids that reduce inflammation and improve the lining of the gut.

Collagen peptides also seem to provide benefits for the immune system by targeting regulatory T (TReg) cells, which help maintain immune balance and prevent autoimmune and inflammatory disorders. The overall impact of collagen peptides appears to be modulation and optimization of redox processes, rather than simply an antioxidant.

## Dosage

Collagen peptides come in powder, capsule, and gummy forms. Recommended dosages vary according to an individual's needs. Most generally, dosages of collagen peptides (as a powder added to a liquid or to soft food) range from 2.5 to 15 g daily. However, refer to the product label and follow the guidelines provided by the manufacturer. Several studies have provided recommendations, such as 2.5 to 10 g daily for skin health over a period of 4 to 12 weeks, or 15 g daily for muscle growth over a period of 12 weeks.

## CREATINE

Creatine is a naturally occurring substance that is synthesized by the body; primarily produced by the pancreas, liver, and kidney; and stored in the cell as phosphocreatine, an energy reserve for muscle cells. Its true power lies in the wide range of benefits it provides for athletes, fitness enthusiasts, and anyone striving for better overall health.

Importantly, creatine acts as a protector of redox balance through adenosine triphosphate (ATP) buffering. After creatine converts into phosphocreatine, it generously donates a phosphate group to adenine dinucleotide phosphate (ADP) to produce ATP, becoming a plentiful source of energy. This buffering action helps maintain ATP levels and acts as a defense against stress that typically accompanies energy depletion.

Creatine has also been associated with brain health. Some studies suggest that creatine may have the potential to enhance cognitive function, including improving memory and attention. Ongoing research is exploring its role in alleviating symptoms of diseases and promoting heart health.

Additionally, creatine possesses antioxidant properties that actively neutralize radicals, protecting our system from oxidative damage. Furthermore, by enhancing nitric oxide (NO) signaling, creatine promotes blood and oxygen flow, preventing stress that may arise due to inadequate oxygen supply (i.e., hypoxia). In general, creatine helps to reduce signals that would otherwise increase oxidative stress and tissue damage.

In addition to boosting muscle strength and power, creatine also enables us to lift more weight and excel at high-intensity exercises. And by enhancing the body's ability to produce energy, creatine extends endurance capacity, reduces fatigue levels, and speeds up recovery time. For those focused on sculpting their physique, creatine helps increase muscle mass by stimulating muscle protein synthesis. Additionally, athletes can take comfort in knowing that creatine may offer an added layer of protection by reducing the risk of injury through its ability to strengthen muscles.

Creatine also helps in the process of methylation, which regulates gene expression by adding a methyl group to DNA, RNA, or proteins governing rhythms from gene expression to metabolism. Specifically, it raises the levels of S-adenosyl methionine (SAM), a methyl donor. Furthermore, creatine acts as a guardian by reducing levels of homocysteine, a non-proteinogenic amino acid known for disrupting methylation and triggering stress and inflammation.

## Dosage

Typically, adults begin with dosages of 2.5 g daily (capsules generally come in 2.5 g). Those using creatine must stay hydrated and consider consuming it along with meals for absorption. The dosage can gradually be increased to 5 g daily.

## EPICATECHIN

Epicatechin, a compound found in cocoa beans, tea leaves, and apples, has been shown to have neuroprotective properties that may reduce the risk of diseases such as Alzheimer's disease and Parkinson's disease. In addition, epicatechin has been found to play an important role in metabolic health because of its help in maintaining blood sugar balance, and it improves blood flow and reduces inflammation, which positions it as a protector of heart health.

Epicatechin, known for its antioxidant properties, plays a role in redox balance because of its ability to fight against reactive oxygen species (ROS). It also boosts the body's natural antioxidant enzymes, such as superoxide dismutase (SOD) and catalase, and it influences signaling pathways related to stress and inflammation. Additionally, by binding to metal ions that contribute to reactions and affecting epigenetic mechanisms that influence gene expression, epicatechin acts as a regulator of cellular health.

By enhancing the body's responsiveness to insulin, epicatechin's anti-inflammatory properties act as a shield against arthritis, asthma, type 2 diabetes, obesity, and cancer. Epicatechin has also been shown to enhance exercise performance by increasing blood flow to muscles and minimizing muscle damage, which leads to increased exercise capacity and endurance.

## Dosage

Proper dosage of epicatechin depends on multiple factors, including age, gender, weight, and overall health. While research often falls within the range of 50 to 1000 mg daily, real-life applications may require some adjustments. For example, in studies focusing on heart health, participants consumed chocolate bars with high epicatechin content, while in studies exploring cognitive function, participants consumed beverages with cocoa flavanols. Another study interested in insulin sensitivity used cocoa drinks with varying levels of epicatechin. Although individual outcomes and reactions differed, the overall conclusion remained consistent: Higher doses of epicatechin generally led to improvements in health. After analyzing the data, it appears that a daily dose ranging from 100 to 1000 mg would be reasonable for a healthy adult seeking to reap the benefits of epicatechin. Epicatechin is best cycled for 3 months on, and then rotated off for 6 weeks.

## KETONE ESTERS

Including ketone esters in one's daily or weekly regimen has been a topic of fascination to many in functional medicine. Ketone esters, which contain molecules of beta-hydroxybutyrate (BHB), help the body produce ketones, which are metabolites that increase energy production and in turn support metabolism and weight loss, enhance athletic performance and recovery, improve cognition and memory, and promote better aging by giving the brain its optimal fuel source.

BHB has control over the instructions within our cells. It inhibits enzymes called *histone deacetylases* and influences the acetylation process of proteins involved in gene expression—both histones and nonhistone proteins are affected. Additionally, BHB can modify protein structures through a process known as *lysine beta-hydroxybutyrylation*. These tuning mechanisms impact the expression of genes such as *FOXO1* and *PPARGC1A*, which are central to metabolism and overall cellular health.

Ketone esters also support redox balance by increasing the availability of nicotinamide adenine dinucleotide (NAD+), a coenzyme that plays a vital role in cellular energy metabolism and redox signaling. Ketone esters can boost NAD+ availability by activating enzymes involved in NAD+ synthesis, such as nicotinamide phosphoribosyltransferase (NAMPT) and nicotinamide riboside kinase (NRK). Ketone esters stimulate these enzymes and thereby reduce oxidative stress. They also increase nicotin-amide adenine dinucleotide phosphate (NADPH), which is important as a master regulator of the antioxidant system.

BHB actively connects to receptors called hydroxycarboxylic acid receptor 2 (HCAR2) and free fatty acid receptors (FFARs) and influences pathways such as NF-κB and cAMP/PKA. When BHB is broken down in the body, it produces coenzyme A (CoA), which increases the ratio of NAD+ to nicotinamide adenine dinucleotide (NADH) and decreases the ratio of NADP to NADPH, thus improving cellular redox. This in turn affects the processes of protein acetylation and succinylation and the functioning of mitochondria, the powerhouses of our cells. One remark-able aspect of ketone metabolism is its efficiency in generating adenos-ine triphosphate (ATP) compared to glucose oxidation. BHB and other ketone bodies enter the tissues, break down to produce acetyl-CoA, and ultimately contribute to ATP production through the acid cycle.

Another interesting aspect of ketone esters is their ability to regulate levels of fatty acids. This regulation might contribute to reducing fatigue. They are also known for their anti-inflammatory properties, potentially providing relief for conditions such as arthritis or even Alzheimer's dis-ease. Additionally, they offer metabolic advantages by helping to reg-ulate blood sugar levels and improving insulin sensitivity, offering a glimmer of hope for individuals dealing with metabolic challenges such as diabetes.

The effects of BHB go beyond our cells. BHB also impacts the com-position of both gut and respiratory microbiota. This ketone body influ-ences mucin secretion and immunoglobulin levels while also helping to modify barrier permeability and junction proteins.

Ketones also offer a strategy for weight loss and metabolic health. Ingesting ketones can elevate insulin levels, a hormone in our metabolic processes. Higher insulin levels can promote increased glucose uptake, which is essential for exercise recovery. Furthermore, the relationship between ketones and the mTOR pathways plays a role in muscle pro-tein synthesis and repair. It seems that ketones can activate these path-ways, emphasizing their role not only in preserving muscles but also in aiding muscle synthesis and repair following intense physical activity.

Supplementing with ketone esters has also been associated with an improvement in cognitive function. Many research studies suggest that ketone esters can improve aspects of cognition, improving attention, processing, and working memory.

For fitness enthusiasts and those interested in endurance activities, ketone esters are believed to enhance endurance by conserving muscle glycogen reserves while promoting the utilization of fatty acids for energy. Another fascinating aspect of ketones is their ability to reduce blood nitrogen levels after exercise, indicating a decrease in protein breakdown, which helps to preserve muscle.

## Dosage

Precision is crucial when it comes to dosing with ketone esters. The ideal dosage depends on factors such as age, weight, metabolic health, and the therapeutic or performance effect being sought. In general, most studies have typically utilized doses ranging from 2.5 to 10 g three times daily. Also available are drinks that come in 12-ounce cans and contain 3 g of ketone esters.

No discussion about ketone supplements would be complete without mentioning ketone salts. Ketone salts cannot be taken more than once daily because of their increased mineral load of sodium, calcium, magnesium, and potassium and their gastrointestinal side effects, which make it difficult to remain in ketosis. Although both are sources of ketones, ketone esters emerge as a more physiological source of ketones because their metabolic pathway ensures a release of ketones into the bloodstream, providing lasting benefits and repetitive use. Ketone salts may only offer a temporary increase in blood ketone levels. Additionally, ketone esters have fewer potential side effects.

## LACTULOSE

Lactulose is a type of carbohydrate (a combination of fructooligosaccharides and galactooligosaccharides) that offers us a powerful prebiotic that promotes the growth and activity of bacteria in the colon. This is the only supplement that is marketed as a synthetic laxative despite it being a prebiotic, and that requires a prescription because of its powerful properties.

Lactulose diversifies the gut microbiota by reducing levels of ammonia, making it an effective detoxifying agent for a host of different conditions, from *Clostridium difficile* to encephalopathy in the brain. When antibiotics and *C. difficile* pose a threat to gut health, lactulose steps up to combat dysbiosis, especially when it's co-administered with antibiotics; it has an ability to restore bacteria in a short period of time, while also facilitating interaction between species through cross feeding. Additionally, lactulose acts as a guardian by inhibiting the growth of bacteria and potential pathogens.

Lactulose stimulates the production of short-chain fatty acids (SCFAs), which are essential for maintaining the health of the gut lining and regulating the immune system by reducing inflammation. For this reason, lactulose has been shown to protect against chronic illnesses such as type 2 diabetes, obesity, and cardiovascular disease by helping to improve cholesterol levels and regulate blood sugar.

It's crucial not to overlook the connection between the gut and mental health. The intricate relationship known as the gut–brain axis is essential for our well-being, and lactulose helps tune this connection by helping to reduce stress and anxiety. Extensive research has also focused on exploring the effects of lactulose on Alzheimer's disease models. The findings were unequivocally impressive: Lactulose effectively protected neurons from beta-amyloid–induced impairments and clearing beta-amyloid from neural pathways. Research also suggests that lactulose can help to reduce memory loss and inflammation in the brain (specifically, astrogliosis within the hippocampus) because it enhances autophagy.

When we delve into the core of neurodegeneration, it becomes clear that chronic inflammation in the brain caused by protein clumps sets the stage for reactive astrogliosis and subsequent neurodegeneration. Lactulose has shown effectiveness in reducing this astrogliosis, indicating its superiority in restoring cognitive function beyond just protecting synapses.

Moreover, lactulose's impact extends to the microorganisms residing in the gut. It notably boosts bacteria populations such as bifidobacteria and increases diversity within the gut microbiota.

Although research on how lactulose influences redox is still in its early stages, initial studies suggest that it plays multiple roles in this area. Lactulose may act as a protector of cells by boosting the production of antioxidants such as glutathione (GSH) and superoxide dismutase (SOD). These antioxidants act as defenders against damage to our cells.

## Dosage

This supplement requires a prescription. Adults generally take 15 to 30 mL (1 to 2 tbsp) daily when using it for constipation relief. For children, doses should be adjusted based on their age and weight. To explore its impact on gut bacteria, studies have examined doses ranging from 7.5 to 30 mL (½ to 2 tbsp) daily.

## L-CARNOSINE

L-carnosine, a dipeptide composed of the amino acids beta-alanine and histidine, naturally exists within the brain and muscle tissues to support their proper functioning, and acts as a shield against various diseases and the natural aging process.

One prominent advantage offered by L-carnosine stems from its antioxidant properties, shielding the cells from stress and damage caused by free radicals. Additionally, L-carnosine possesses the ability to bind to metals such as copper and iron, which can generate radicals while contributing to stress. This is not merely a strategy; it represents an approach to preventing disease and slowing down the aging process. Furthermore, L-carnosine acts as a nourishing tonic for the brain by alleviating brain fog, sharpening focus, and potentially reducing the risk of neurodegenerative conditions such as Alzheimer's disease and Parkinson's disease.

Our eyes, often considered the window to our soul, also receive support and protection, as this compound has shown potential in safeguarding against conditions such as cataracts by reducing stress and inflammation in the eyes.

Delving deeper, L-carnosine inhibits cellular senescence, which refers to a cell's progression toward retirement, by combating the inflammatory responses that exacerbate senescence and trigger diseases. Specifically, it has an inhibitory effect on mTor, the TGF/Smad-3 pathway, and an antioxidant and anti-glycation effect. L-carnosine also helps the body's immune system by improving autophagy, ensuring that our cells remain clean and efficient as we age. L-carnosine has a significant antiglycation effect; it has been found to suppress glycation by 42% and reduce advanced glycation end products (AGE) by 70%. L-carnosine is more potent than L-carnitine, whose effect is minimal.

L-carnosine reduces wrinkles and fine lines and strengthens our immune system by enhancing blood cell activity and improving our ability to fight infections. For athletes and fitness enthusiasts, it has demonstrated an ability to reduce muscle fatigue and increase endurance.

## Dosage

While the advantages of L-carnosine seem limitless, it's important to note that determining the dosage is an area of active research. For improving overall health while aging, the typical recommended dosage is 500 to 1500 mg divided into two or three doses over the course of 1 day. Athletes may consider increased amounts, but levels should be increased gradually. L-carnosine comes in capsule and powder forms. This supplement is best used in a cycle of 3 months on, 6 weeks off.

## L-CITRULLINE

L-citrulline is a naturally occurring amino acid that has been shown to nurture the heart and circulatory system by helping to regulate blood pressure and improve circulation. By increasing blood flow and promoting nitric oxide production, it can elevate workouts and help athletes reach new heights while reducing fatigue, alleviating muscle soreness, and speeding up recovery.

L-citrulline boosts energy levels by promoting the production of adenosine triphosphate (ATP), the source of cellular energy in the body. Additionally, L-citrulline supports redox balance: As it transforms into L-arginine within the body, it facilitates the production of nitric oxide (which is essential for redox balance) by eliminating oxygen species and ensures that cells function optimally. The body has the ability to absorb L-citrulline quickly and retain it for periods (compared to L-arginine, for instance). Interestingly, L-citrulline supplements can increase arginine levels.

While excessive doses of L-arginine can disrupt the system and lead to issues such as diarrhea, L-citrulline remains harmless, with no side effects. However, it's important to note that L-citrulline and L-arginine are not in competition; they can coexist harmoniously as supplements, each enhancing the effects of the other.

L-citrulline also acts as an inhibitor of inflammatory pathways such as NF-κB and mitogen-activated protein kinase (MAPK), offering hope to those fighting inflammation. L-citrulline supports mitochondria growth while reducing the production of oxygen species. The result is a strengthened environment that is better protected against stress. Additionally, this amino acid plays a role in safeguarding DNA by enhancing DNA repair mechanisms and maintaining the integrity of the DNA blueprint.

## Dosage

In general, I recommend taking 1.5 to 6 g daily, in divided doses (powder or capsule). Those seeking peak exercise performance can benefit from an intake of 6 to 8 g distributed throughout the day.

## LITHIUM OROTATE

Low-dose lithium orotate has been shown to offer a range of health benefits, including enhancing heart function, bone density and reformation, blood sugar regulation, the microbiome, and especially mental health.

In terms of balancing redox, low-dose lithium helps to reduce oxidative stress and inflammation by inhibiting pathways and enhancing antioxidant activity in the body. Exciting research has recently surfaced indicating that even small doses of lithium may also have positive effects on kidney health. Studies conducted on fruit flies and *Caenorhabditis elegans* (nematodes) have demonstrated that lithium can extend lifespan and slow down brain aging. These findings hold implications for how we approach aging in humans.

Research has also shown that low-dose lithium inhibits the activity of an enzyme called *GSK3*, which in turn boosts the effectiveness of SERCA, a protein for calcium transport within heart cells. This improved cardiac output may also play a role in reducing the risk of atherosclerosis by lowering levels of VCAM-1, a protein that facilitates blood cell adhesion to blood vessel walls.

Low-dose lithium has been associated with the stimulation of bone formation and increased bone density through the activation of Wnt–beta catenin signaling pathways. These pathways play a role in promoting the growth and healing processes within our bone tissue. Lithium may also have positive effects on muscle performance, potentially influencing the types of muscle fibers that improve endurance and resistance against fatigue. The Wnt–beta cantenin pathway is disrupted in Parkinson's disease and inhibited by GFK 3. Low-dose lithium has the potential to inhibit GKF 3.

For individuals dealing with metabolic challenges such as diabetes and obesity, animal studies have shown that low-dose lithium can lower blood glucose levels and enhance energy expenditure by improving insulin sensitivity.

One area of research that holds promise is the use of low-dose lithium in reducing the accumulation of beta-amyloid plaques and tau tangles, both features of Alzheimer's disease. By inhibiting GSK3, an enzyme involved in the development of these conditions, lithium could potentially safeguard brain function. Preliminary evidence from studies including an analysis conducted by the University of Cambridge indicates a potential decrease in dementia risk among older adults who have used low-dose lithium. While larger studies are needed to confirm these findings, they provide encouraging insights into the role of lithium in preventing decline. Unlike lithium-based medications, which can come with side effects, low-dose lithium supplements are emerging as a gentler alternative to help balance mood and alleviate feelings of anxiety and irritability that many individuals experience. Although there is no contraindication in the use of low-dose lithium and antidepressants such as selective serotonin reuptake inhibitors (SSRIs), patients should consult their healthcare provider when introducing this supplement.

## Dosage

When it comes to supplementing with lithium orotate, the recommended daily dosage can range from 5 to 20 mg.

## L-LEUCINE

L-leucine is an essential branched-chain amino acid that the body cannot produce naturally, so we must obtain it through our diet or supplements. L-leucine is found in a variety of foods, including meat, poultry, fish, eggs, and dairy products. L-leucine is also found in plant-based foods such as soybeans, lentils, peas, quinoa, and nuts. Additionally, for those who prefer other options, protein supplements such as whey protein isolate can be a source.

At its core, L-leucine supports cellular redox by promoting the activity of antioxidant defense enzymes such as superoxide dismutase (SOD) and catalase. SOD acts as a hero enzyme that combats radicals by transforming them into harmful substances that are then detoxified by catalase or glutathione peroxidase. Furthermore, L-leucine boosts the production of glutathione (GSH)—a superstar in our body—by increasing the availability of cysteine, which is necessary for GSH synthesis. This protects cells from damage caused by oxidation, which ensures their well-being and longevity.

L-leucine plays a role in weight loss and promotes an increase in muscle mass while simultaneously reducing body fat. Another advantage is its ability to regulate blood sugar levels and control appetite, making it easier to stick to calorie-restricted diets. Additionally, L-leucine plays a role in strengthening the immune system and enhances the body's ability to defend against infections and diseases. Moreover, it contributes significantly to maintaining bone health, reducing the risk of conditions such as osteoporosis.

It also serves as a foundation for muscle growth and repair; stimulates the body's ability to build muscle mass; and enhances exercise performance by increasing endurance, reducing fatigue, and expediting post-workout muscle recovery. This can aid in making workout sessions more intense, last longer, and yield results. Lastly, low-dose leucine (around 1 gram) enhances availability of NAD+ to activate SIRT 1. It can also enhance the NAD+ salvage pathway by increasing the rate-limiting enzyme nicotinamide phosphoribosyltransferase, which produces more NAD+.

## Dosage

The types of benefits of L-leucine can vary depending on dosage. When taken in doses of approximately 1.6 to 3 g (capsule or powder), L-leucine moderately stimulates muscle protein synthesis while assisting in weight loss and supporting bone and immune health. Doses exceeding 2.5 g can help to increase muscle growth, improve bone density, and increase exercise endurance.

Optimal dosage is dependent on the individual. Research emphasizes that consuming around 2 to 3 g of L-leucine is necessary to optimize muscle protein synthesis. Nevertheless, the synergistic effects with acids or protein sources may make even lower doses effective when combined with resistance exercises. Individual needs may dictate the optimal amount. When you're sipping on the Amino Drink all day, you are benefiting from the effects of low-dose L-leucine.

## L-THEANINE

L-theanine, an amino acid found in tea leaves, is an incredible compound that promotes relaxation without causing drowsiness. As a natural antianxiety substance, it helps alleviate stress and anxiety by boosting alpha waves in the brain—a state associated with tranquility and calmness. At the same time, L-theanine also leads to improved focus and concentration.

In terms of supporting redox, L-theanine possesses powerful antioxidant properties that can help reduce stress within the cells. While researchers are still uncovering the details about how it works, a few things are clear: L-theanine increases the production of the antioxidant glutathione (GSH), which neutralizes reactive oxygen species (ROS) and makes them harmless; and it activates antioxidant enzymes such as superoxide dismutase (SOD), which further strengthens the cells' defense against oxidative stress. Some studies suggest that L-theanine can lower ROS production altogether. And let's not forget its role in regulating signaling pathways such as the NRF2 pathway; this highlights its potential for enhancing redox balance.

Additionally, L-theanine strengthens the production of specific immune cells that reduce inflammation. An interesting study showed that combining L-theanine with catechins decreased symptoms of influenza. This positive outcome was attributed to an improvement in gamma-delta T-cell proliferation and an increase in interferon-gamma secretion. Another intriguing study found that post-exercise supplementation of L-theanine resulted in a decrease in IL10 concentration accompanied by levels of Th1 cytokines. However, it's important to note that without stimulation, substantial concentrations of alkylamines are required to induce gamma-delta T-cell proliferation. While current findings are promising regarding L-theanine, its influence on the immune system requires further rigorous research to determine its effect on gamma-delta T cells.

L-theanine may also improve sleep quality. By increasing the production of gamma-aminobutyric acid (GABA), a neurotransmitter associated with relaxation and sleep, L-theanine promotes deep sleep. And for females, L-theanine seems to ease the symptoms of premenstrual syndrome, such as irritability, bloating, and unexpected mood swings. Further, research suggests that this amino acid has shown promise in supporting heart health by regulating blood pressure levels and improving profiles.

## Dosing

When it comes to dosing, it's crucial to consider factors such as age, weight, and overall health. Most studies investigating the effects of L-theanine suggest a range of 100 to 400 mg daily, either taken at once or divided into two doses. Some research even delved into amounts of up to 600 mg daily without observing any negative side effects. The good news is that L-theanine is generally considered safe and well tolerated at these doses. L-theanine is available in capsule and powder forms. L-theanine is best used in rotation: 3 months on, 6 weeks off.

## L-TRYPTOPHAN

L-tryptophan, an essential amino acid that we can get from food sources or as a supplement, helps to regulate mood because it acts as a building block for serotonin, the neurotransmitter closely associated with emotion regulation as well as the regulation of appetite and sleep. Raising L-tryptophan levels has been shown to reduce symptoms of depression and anxiety. Given its role in the production of neurotransmitters such as serotonin and dopamine, research suggests that L-tryptophan could also benefit individuals with mild cognitive impairments. It's also connected to melatonin, a hormone that helps regulate sleep patterns. In addition, for females, L-tryptophan has been shown to relieve the symptoms of premenstrual syndrome such as mood swings, irritability, and intense food cravings. It also possesses anti-inflammatory properties.

L-tryptophan helps increase the production of glutathione (GSH), an antioxidant derived from amino acids, thereby supporting redox balance. This increased production strengthens cells against the damaging effects of stress. Interestingly, L-tryptophan's ability to activate the NRF2 pathway further enhances defense mechanisms, forming a shield against potential harm to cells. It also helps inhibit the creation of reactive oxygen species (ROS) that cause cell damage. Additionally, its connection to the kynurenine pathway suggests that L-tryptophan may have the potential to reduce the production of metabolites while promoting the generation of neuroprotective ones.

Some initial research suggests that infections caused by viruses such as COVID-19 cause a decrease in tryptophan levels. This depletion could hinder the recovery process and increase the risk of long-term effects of COVID-19. Also fascinating is how L-tryptophan converts into serotonin. In people suffering from the long-term effects of COVID-19, serotonin levels are reduced, potentially explaining why sufferers experience depressed mood, memory problems, and loss of some cognitive functions.

## Dosage

Like any supplement, proper dosage is vital. The appropriate amount of L-tryptophan depends on factors such as age and overall health status. For adults, the recommended dosage typically falls within the range of 1 to 3 g daily, divided into three or four doses. In some cases, specific conditions may require doses of up to 6 g daily. High doses can lead to side effects such as drowsiness or gastrointestinal (GI) issues. It is crucial that patients on other medications consult their healthcare specialist due to interactions of this substance with medications, particularly antidepressants and antianxiety drugs. L-tryptophan is best rotated: on for 3 months, off for 6 weeks.

# OLIVE LEAF EXTRACT

Derived from the olive tree, olive leaf extract is an interesting supplement, one that is a bridge between traditional wisdom and modern scientific knowledge. Ancient civilizations have long revered the olive's properties, and current research only reinforces the power of olive leaf extract as it contains numerous antioxidants that protect against overall inflammation.

Studies have shown that this supplement protects against heart disease, alleviates chronic inflammatory conditions such as type 2 diabetes, boosts production of blood cells, and restrains the growth of cancer cells. As such, it contains powerful antimicrobial capabilities that fight against bacteria, viruses, and fungi. Further, olive leaf extract supports redox balance by enhancing the activity of antioxidant enzymes such as superoxide dismutase (SOD) and catalase. This ensures that harmful radicals are efficiently converted into substances that preserve the integrity of cells.

The relationship between olive leaf extract and thyroid function is an interplay of biochemistry. The balance of thyroid hormones is maintained through the conversion of T4 to T3 at the periphery. However, oxidative stress and inflammation can disrupt this equilibrium. This is where olive leaf extract comes into play. Numerous studies have shown the remarkable capabilities of olive leaf extract to help convert thyroid hormones in peripheral areas (converting T4 to T3) and help manage subclinical hypothyroidism, a condition in which patients experience symptoms such as fatigue, weight gain, and intolerance to cold.

## Dosage

The recommended dosage can vary depending on the product, form, and intended use. Most studies suggest a daily dose ranging from 500 to 1000 mg. However, it's important to remember that while research provides some guidance, personalization is key. Products are also available in dosages of 250 to 400 mg. I recommend rotating this supplement: 3 months on, 6 weeks off.

## OMEGA-3 FATTY ACIDS

Omega-3 fatty acids, including eicosapentaenoic acid (EPA) and docosahexaenoic acid (DHA), are vital polyunsaturated fatty acids that help maintain redox balance. Although we can obtain omega-3s from sources such as fish, flaxseeds, and walnuts, we often don't get enough to benefit our health. Indeed, consuming omega-3 supplements has been shown to help with glucose metabolism, improve insulin sensitivity, and lower resting blood glucose levels. Additionally, omega-3s offer protection against a range of diseases including cardiac issues, metabolic disorders, neurodegenerative conditions, and visual impairments. In older individuals, omega-3s can help preserve muscles and fight sarcopenia.

Omega-3 and omega-6 are crucial for the body's well-being, but because our body is unable to produce enough omega-3 and omega-6 on its own, we need to obtain them from outside sources. However, the Western diet often has an excess of omega-6 (from vegetable oils) and a deficiency of omega-3 (from fish and plants). This imbalance can result in inflammation.

Omega-3s also improve energy through a process called beta-oxidation and help to resolve inflammation and promote tissue repair. I believe this is one of the most underestimated benefits of omega-3 fatty acids and is crucial to cellular redox.

One way in which omega-3 fatty acids contribute to redox is by replacing arachidonic acid in the membranes of our cells. Various studies have demonstrated that when we absorb EPA and DHA, these fatty acids are incorporated into cell membranes effectively. This replacement of arachidonic acid helps ensure an interplay between oxidants and anti-oxidants within our cells.

Omega-3s play a crucial role in resolving inflammation; they serve as precursors to resolvins,  protectins, maresins, and lytoxsins—otherwise known as pro-resolvins. The inability to resolve inflammation has played a significant role in chronic problems secondary to SARS COVID-19 exposure and vaccination.

To evaluate whether someone is getting enough supplementation with omega-3 fatty acids, I would suggest having them take an Omega-3 Index test, which evaluates the levels of EPA and DHA in the bloodstream and membranes of blood cells. It is a validated indicator of health and is expressed as a percentage. An ideal Omega-3 Index is considered to be 8% or higher, indicating a low risk zone for coronary heart disease (CHD); a level below 4% is associated with a high risk zone. This test only requires a drop of blood and provides valuable information about an individual's omega-3 status. With over 200 studies supporting its use and standardized procedures over time, the Omega-3 Index test has become a reliable tool for monitoring overall health.

## Dosage

According to the Harvard T.H. Chan School of Public Health, incorporating fish into the diet twice weekly could potentially lower the risk of stroke, depression, Alzheimer's disease, and other chronic conditions.

The Mayo Clinic also suggests including at least two servings of fish weekly to help reduce the risk of heart disease. The American Heart Association advises consuming two servings of fish (3 ounces cooked, or about ¾ cup) weekly, with an emphasis on fatty fish such as salmon, mackerel, and sardines due to their high omega-3 fatty acid content.

If choosing supplementation, I prefer to use a phospholipid source such as krill oil, ingesting between 1 and 2 g daily (capsule form). It's important to pay attention to manufacturing standards and potential oxidation of omega-3 supplements. Many omega-3 supplements (70% of 45 brands) do not contain the stated dose of EPA and DHA due to variations in manufacturing standards. Further, over 80% of 35 brands had high levels of oxidized lipids, indicating lipid degradation. The reason I recommend phospholipid is for improved brain absorption; clinical research shows it crosses the blood–brain barrier with better results.

## PENTADECANOIC ACID

Pentadecanoic acid (C15:0) is a naturally occurring odd-chain saturated fatty acid that can be found in small amounts in dairy foods, certain fish species, and plants and is now recognized as a fatty acid that's necessary to support overall physiological health. Although there has been an emphasis on the dangers of dairy intake, dairy remains a good source of pentadecanoic acid, which not only plays a crucial role in maintaining cellular redox balance and enhancing mitochondrial function but is seen by researchers as having broad implications in cancer prevention, cardiac health, immune health, and liver functioning.

Research has demonstrated the importance of pentadecanoic acid in acting as an antioxidant and providing essential fatty acids and substrates necessary for maintaining cellular health. Pentadecanoic acid, as an essential fatty acid, plays a crucial role in maintaining cellular redox and mitochondrial efficiency. One study demonstrated that pure C15:0 rescues mitochondrial function at complex II of the mitochondrial respiratory pathway by increasing the production of succinate, a key component involved in cellular respiration and energy production.

The study suggests that the presence of pentadecanoic acid enhances mitochondrial efficiency and contributes to improved cellular function.

Pentadecanoic acid activates AMP-activated protein kinase (AMPK), which is involved in regulating cellular energy homeostasis, and it inhibits mTOR, a key regulator of cell growth and metabolism. Both AMPK and mTOR are core components of the human longevity pathway. Pentadecanoic acid also acts as a substrate for the synthesis of coenzyme A (CoA). CoA is a critical molecule involved in several metabolic pathways, including fatty acid beta-oxidation and energy production. By providing the necessary precursor, pentadecanoic acid ensures the efficient production of CoA, which supports the antioxidant system and contributes to the regulation of apoptosis in response to stress-inducing or regulatory signals. This indicates that pentadecanoic acid may protect cells from oxidative stress and promote cell survival.

Additionally, pentadecanoic acid serves as a substrate for the synthesis of important cellular components such as membrane phospholipids and sphingolipids. These lipids are crucial for maintaining the integrity and fluidity of cellular membranes as well as for various signaling processes within cells.

Orally administered C15:0 can improve red blood cell stability, attenuate anemia, and reduce liver iron deposition. Recently, C15:0 is being utilized as a broad chemotherapy treatment for various types of cancer, including those of the breast, lung, ovary, and pancreas. The use of pentadecanoic acid in combination with other drugs, such as gemcitabine and paclitaxel, has been shown to enhance the effectiveness of chemotherapy in some cases. Research has also identified pentadecanoic acid as a potential therapeutic agent for targeting the stemness in tumors, which is a promising strategy for developing novel cancer treatments. In breast cancer cells, pentadecanoic acid has been found to serve as a JAK2/STAT3 signaling inhibitor, suppressing the stemness of cancer stemlike cells. Another study suggests that it may enhance the efficacy of endocrine therapy in the treatment of ER-alpha-underexpressing breast cancer.

# Dosing

Typical dosing is 100 mg (capsule) daily to maintain adequate serum levels for producing positive redox effects. Although we do get some amount of pentadecanoic acid in serum either by conversions of other fatty acids or by diet, I believe supplementation ensures a physiological level of the odd-chain fatty acid that is needed to ensure a better oxidative state. I also believe this odd-chain fatty acid **coupled** with a phospholipid source of omega-3 is very important in maintaining optimal fatty acid metabolism and ultimate cellular redox. You need both of these because they have different mechanisms for improving cellular health.

## PLASMALOGENS

Found in concentrations within brain tissue, plasmalogens are remarkable phospholipids that are abundant in photoreceptor cells of the eye and have been shown to have a very positive impact on cognitive function. Numerous studies have shed light on a concerning association between low levels of plasmalogens and cognitive decline, even suggesting a heightened risk for conditions such as Alzheimer's disease. However, with supplementation, you can achieve protective mechanisms against neurodegenerative conditions such as Alzheimer's disease as well as cardiovascular disorders.

These molecules diligently protect the heart by reducing inflammation, improving blood lipid profiles, and shielding the heart from stress; they also protect against macular degeneration. Although they contain a vinyl ether bond that unfortunately makes them vulnerable to oxidation, they counteract this vulnerability by acting as antioxidants, playing a role in maintaining the balance of cellular redox. They effectively combat reactive oxygen species (ROS), regulate the expression of antioxidant enzymes, and modulate signaling pathways related to redox sensitivity, such as NF-κB, mitogen-activated protein kinase (MAPK), and PPAR pathways.

At the core of several methylation processes, in particular in the synthesis of S-adenosyl methionine (SAM), is a molecule for providing methyl groups. These methyl groups are essential for reactions that occur within cells. Plasmalogens serve as a source of choline, which is necessary for the synthesis of SAM. By promoting the production and breakdown of plasmalogens, we indirectly impact the levels of SAM in our body, ensuring progress in methylation reactions.

Plasmalogens also influence proper DNA methylation, a process that controls gene expression through modifications. In this capacity, plasmalogens also affect DNA methyltransferases (DNMTs), which are enzymes responsible for transferring methyl groups from SAM to DNA. Studies suggest that plasmalogens play a role in inhibiting activity leading to reduced DNA methylation levels and triggering significant changes in gene expression patterns with potential implications for overall health.

Our diet offers a source of plasmalogens in animal-based products. Seafood such as fatty fish and shellfish are abundant in plasmalogens. Meat and dairy also provide phospholipids. However, it's important to note that factors such as food processing and dietary choices can impact the levels of plasmalogens in our food sources, and for individuals with reduced levels or metabolic impairments, supplementation may be necessary to access the benefits of plasmalogens.

## Dosage

Plasmalogen supplements are available in capsule and liquid forms. My patients take from 900 to 3600 mg daily, with a typical patient taking 1800 to 2700 mg daily.

While some studies have explored dosage ranges, extensive human trials are required to determine an ideal dose that fully unlocks the potential of plasmalogens. Most studies investigating plasmalogen supplementation have been carried out on animals or in laboratory settings. The dosages used in these studies vary significantly. Certain clinical trials have explored the impact of plasmalogen supplementation on health conditions such as Alzheimer's disease and cardiovascular disease using doses that range from 0.6 to 2 g daily.

# SPERMIDINE

Spermidine is a post-biotic produced in the microbiome. This remarkable polyamine has been shown to support cognition and fight against cognitive decline associated with Alzheimer's disease, lower blood pressure, improve blood circulation, and reduce the risk of heart disease. In the case of dysbiosis, the body will not be able to produce this important metabolite. This longevity supplement, taken in capsule form, supports the immune system's function of autophagy, eliminating damaged cells and waste. Its anti-inflammatory properties suggest that it can help to lower the risk of illnesses such as cancer and diabetes, promote hair growth, and improve skin.

Through mechanisms and its impact on cellular pathways, spermidine improves redox balance by reducing the production of oxygen species that contribute to oxidative stress. Spermidine not only has antioxidant properties that effectively scavenge free radicals, but it also promotes the growth of functional mitochondria within cells. Spermidine also regulates gene expression through mechanisms such as histone acetylation and DNA methylation and the activation of the NRF2 pathway, vital for managing stress and further solidifying its role in maintaining redox balance.

## Dosage

For those considering incorporating spermidine into their health routine, typical doses range from 800 to 2500 mg daily (capsule). As a polyamine, spermidine can be found in legumes such as soybeans, lentils, peas, and chickpeas. Additionally, whole grains such as wheat, rye, and oats contain this compound. Mushrooms including shiitake, portobello, and white button are all sources of spermidine. Similarly, fruits such as grapefruit, oranges, strawberries, and kiwis as well as cruciferous vegetables such as broccoli, cauliflower, spinach, and asparagus contain spermidine. Certain types of hard cheese (e.g., cheddar), blue cheese, and organ meats (e.g., beef liver and chicken liver) also contain spermidine. When taking spermidine as a supplement, I recommend rotating 3 months on, 6 weeks off.

# SPIRULINA

Spirulina, an algae with a blue-green hue, has captivated the health community for its outstanding nutritional value. It is a rich source of plant protein that is packed with a variety of vitamins, minerals, and antioxidants. Whether you're looking for a source of iron, calcium, magnesium, potassium, or vitamins B and K, spirulina has you covered. This intriguing algae has the potential to support the system to such an extent that it can ward off types of cancer.

This algae powerhouse contains phycocyanin, a protein known for its immunity-boosting properties and ability to reduce inflammation. Research suggests that spirulina may play a role in lowering cholesterol levels and improving insulin sensitivity, which helps maintain stable blood sugar levels. Phycocyanin neutralizes free radicals and reactive oxygen species (ROS) and transforms superoxide radicals into less damaging hydrogen peroxide. Spirulina also triggers the activation of a bioavailable superoxide dismutase (SOD). Together, these features boost glutathione (GSH), which protects cells, and activates the NRF2 pathway, which helps regulate the expression of antioxidant enzymes and other protective genes, ensuring the health and balance of our cells.

Spirulina acts as a weapon against stress due to its antioxidant properties. Furthermore, spirulina's ability to reduce inflammation adds another layer of benefit. Since chronic inflammation can lead to the production of ROS that cause damage, spirulina's anti-inflammatory properties indirectly support cellular redox.

Research also suggests that spirulina may enhance muscle strength and endurance. Additionally, for those seeking weight loss, spirulina has been shown to reduce appetite and promote a feeling of fullness.

## Dosage

Finding the dosage for spirulina can be a bit challenging. Whether it is ingested in tablet or powder form, there are some guidelines to follow. The National Institutes of Health (NIH) recommends doses of up to 19 g daily for a period of 2 months and up to 10 g daily for up to 12 months. However, it's important to note that there isn't an absolute recommended dose for spirulina use. The specific dosages vary depending on the condition for which it is used. For instance, for managing cholesterol levels, doses ranging from 1 to 8 g daily can have a positive impact.

I typically recommend that patients take 3 g daily. For enhancing muscle performance, doses between 2 and 7.5 g daily have been utilized. It's worth noting that spirulina acts as a cleanser and aids in eliminating toxins from the body during the initial consumption phase. Some individuals may experience changes in their digestive system during the first few days of taking spirulina. Therefore, it is recommended to start with a small dosage and gradually increase it over time. Taken as a supplement, spirulina should be rotated: 3 months on, 6 weeks off.

## SYTRINOL

Sytrinol is a capsule supplement made from a blend of citrus and palm fruit extracts that targets cholesterol—reducing LDL ("bad" cholesterol) and boosting HDL ("good" cholesterol) levels in the blood. Sytrinol also contains anti-inflammatory properties and is rich in antioxidants that fight against free radical damage.

Packed with antioxidants such as flavonoids, polymethoxylated flavones (PMFs) such as tangeretins and nobilitans, and tocotrienols (isomers of vitamin E), sytrinol contributes to improving redox balance. Its ability to both lower LDL levels and fight against free radicals decreases oxidative stress and supports overall cellular health, including acting as a nutrient for the microbiome, and it contributes to SIRT-1 activation, which is important to mitochondrial health and redox balance. Research also suggests that sytrinol could help balance blood sugar levels and safeguard against diabetes and other metabolic disorders. At a deeper level, researchers have also shown that sytrinol possesses the ability to regulate the expression of genes associated with cholesterol metabolism. This unique capability demonstrates its effectiveness in lowering cholesterol levels.

Because of its cholesterol-lowering effects, sytrinol is positioned to be a potentially healthier option than statins to lower cholesterol. One study drew similarities between sytrinol and atorvastatin, revealing that both were successful in lowering cholesterol levels without any difference in their efficacy. Another study compared sytrinol to simvastatin with regard to stress and inflammation. In this case, sytrinol not only matched the ability of the statin to reduce lipid levels and oxidative stress markers, but outperformed it by significantly reducing inflammation markers. (My recommendation regarding sytrinol is not meant as a suggestion that you give up statins; please consult your physician before making any changes.)

## Dosage

For those incorporating sytrinol (capsule form) into their routine, the recommended daily dosage generally ranges from 300 to 600 mg divided into two or three doses and taken with meals for optimal results.

## TREHALOSE

Trehalose is a form of natural sugar that works very differently than the common form of sugar, known as sucrose, which is a type of disaccharide made from the combination of the monosaccharides glucose and fructose.

Though a disaccharide, trehalose interacts with water differently, enabling it to actively enhance the integrity of the gut barrier by increasing the expression of junction proteins. These proteins act as guardians for the gut, ensuring that harmful substances are prevented from breaching the barrier and causing inflammation in the bloodstream. At the forefront of this defense mechanism in the gut, specifically related to the associated lymphoid tissue galactose-1-phosphate uridyl transferase (GALT), trehalose helps to both repel pathogens and regulate immune responses. In this function, trehalose strengthens GALT's capabilities, thereby bolstering our defenses. Further, trehalose acts like a gardener, carefully nurturing the growth of bacteria such as bifidobacteria and lactobacillus. Simultaneously, it keeps strains in check, creating a balanced and harmonious environment within the gut.

Trehalose interacts with glucose transport in a few ways. First, it decreases glucose absorption within the intestine and counteracts an excessive production of insulin, reinforcing its capacity to help regulate blood sugar levels. And further, it enhances insulin sensitivity, a factor when it comes to preventing and managing diabetes.

Trehalose has been observed to stimulate autophagy and greatly reduce levels of oxygen species, which cause cellular damage. By increasing the expression of genes such as *PGC-1alpha* and *NRF1*, which are involved in biogenesis, trehalose promotes the creation and optimal functioning of mitochondria, which improves overall energy production and function. By actively engaging with AMP-activated protein kinase (AMPK), trehalose not only helps manage cellular energy but also triggers autophagy, which is crucial for energy and mitochondrial regulation and efficiency.

Trehalose influences gene expression related to energy metabolism and mitochondrial functions involved in fatty acid oxidation and glucose dynamics. Further studies have shed light on the role of trehalose in combating disorders such as Alzheimer's disease and Parkinson's disease. By reducing the buildup of proteins in the brain, trehalose acts as a guardian for neural pathways. Moreover, it exhibits an ability to enhance cell survival in challenging conditions such as dehydration, extreme temperatures, and nutrient scarcity—all factors that can make the brain vulnerable to disease. Because of trehalose's capacity to activate autophagy, it may mitigate the devastating effects of neurodegenerative disorders.

Additionally, researchers are closely observing the role of trehalose in the field of oncology. It has shown promise in inhibiting tumor growth and enhancing the effectiveness of chemotherapy drugs. As we age, our liver's metabolic function undergoes disruptions that increase the risk for liver conditions and other systemic diseases. Trehalose has gained attention for its potential to mitigate age-related challenges such as dyslipidemia, hepatic steatosis, and glucose intolerance.

Athletes and fitness enthusiasts may benefit from trehalose's capacity to grow muscle mass and strength.

## Dosage

In general, I recommend supplementing with trehalose at 2 to 4 scoops (5 g/scoop) daily. Most of my patients add it to their morning coffee, tea, or other drink of choice. For individuals who tend to have elevated post-meal glucose levels within the normal range, incorporating a daily intake of 3.3 g of trehalose for 78 days has shown promising effects in reducing these spikes. (I recommend 1 or 2 scoops (5–10 g) at the beginning of each meal.) This moderate amount can easily be included in meals. However, for a more therapeutic dose to address blood sugar balance, a study showed that a daily intake of 10 g of trehalose improved glucose tolerance and slowed down the progression of insulin resistance. Those interested in boosting athletic performance might consider supplementing in the range of 20 to 40 g daily.

## TUDCA

TUDCA, or tauroursodeoxycholic acid, is a naturally occurring bile acid post-biotic that functions as both an antioxidant and an ally for mito-chondria. By enhancing the function of bile acid, TUDCA enables cells to operate more efficiently while at the same time actively combating inflammation in the body.

TUDCA is especially supportive to the liver's detoxification processes, as well as offering overall brain protection. In addition to its known functions in aiding lipid absorption in the intestines and regulating cholesterol levels, TUDCA has been recognized for its hormone-signaling abilities. This signaling plays a role in biological processes, particularly neurological well-being. Recent research emphasizes the connection between the gut microbiome and the brain—an association often referred to as the gut–brain axis. Within this axis, bile acid–mediated signaling seems to be bidirectional, affecting metabolic status and cholesterol balance within the nervous system. It is concerning to note that brains affected by diseases often show high levels of secondary bile acids. This increase could be due to an imbalance in the gut microbiome leading to production of bile acids. Elevated levels of bile acids in the bloodstream can also pose risks by affecting the permeability of the blood–brain barrier.

TUDCA effectively enhances redox status through various molecular pathways, including the NRF2 pathway, which is important to our cellular antioxidant defense system. Its activation leads to increased expression of antioxidant enzymes, providing even greater protection against oxidative stress. Furthermore, TUDCA helps maintain balance by inhibiting reticulum (ER) stress and preventing excessive production of reactive oxygen species (ROS) that can harm cells. Moreover, by regulating the function of mitochondria and reducing inflammation, TUDCA ensures that cellular redox balance remains in harmony.

TUDCA is synthesized by the liver through the combination of taurine, an amino acid, and ursodeoxycholic acid, which is found in the gut. Importantly, hydrophilic bile acids such as TUDCA have the ability to cross the blood–brain barrier and act as agonists for bile acid receptors, enabling them to protect brain health.

## Dosage

My general recommendation is 500 mg daily (capsule); however, dosages can vary depending on factors such as age, weight, and specific health conditions. For example, individuals with liver disease may require doses ranging from 500 to 2000 mg daily. For people who suffer from disorders such as Alzheimer's disease, doses range from 500 to 1200 mg daily. It is important to note that the effectiveness of TUDCA also depends on its purity and the quality of the supplement itself. TUDCA is best used in rotation: 3 months on, 6 weeks off.

## UROLITHIN A

Urolithin A, a metabolite of ellagic acid that is also a post-biotic, can be ingested from certain nuts, berries, and fruit such as pomegranates. Urolithin A has been found to have significant anti-inflammatory properties, improve mitochondrial health, and increase muscle function—all of which support better aging.

Urolithin A is not found in food directly, but rather is produced when ellagic acid and ellagitannins are metabolized by gut bacteria in the body. Although foods such as pomegranates can help the gut microflora convert ellagic acid into usable urolithin A, most people lack the gut microbiome diversity needed to produce adequate amounts of urolithin A from dietary sources alone. Urolithin A may improve health by reducing ceramide levels and inflammation. Ceramides are a class of sphingolipids (waxy lipid molecules) linked to inflammation and age-associated diseases. Indeed, accumulation of ceramide is associated with cardiovascular diseases and several age-associated diseases such as Alzheimer's disease and diabetes. Studies suggest that supplementing with urolithin A reduces ceramide levels, specifically levels of C16 and C18 ceramides. Other research has shown that urolithin A may offer a potential treatment for muscular dystrophy.

Recent animal and human studies have pointed to the following important health benefits from supplementing with urolithin A:

- Improves mitochondrial and cellular health
- Exhibits anti-inflammatory properties in cells and animal models
- Increases muscle function in rodent models
- Increases mitochondrial biogenesis (i.e., growth of new mitochondria)
- Activates mitophagy (i.e., removal of old and damaged mitochondria)
- Inhibits NF-kB signaling, which decreases inflammation

## Dosage

The typical and standard dosing we use for urolithin A is 500 mg daily. On average, the normal range is 250 to 500 mg, with 500 mg as standard across the board. In recent studies, 500 mg daily for 6 weeks decreased inflammatory markers in obese adults. In another study, 500 mg daily for 4 weeks improved markers of muscle function in older adults. The conclusion of a study comparing supplementation versus ingesting ellagic acid through food determined that direct urolithin A supplementation provides more consistent levels of urolithin A compared to pomegranate juice, overcoming microbiome limitations; only 40% of people can naturally produce urolithin A from pomegranate juice due to gut microbiome composition. Urolithin A is best rotated: 3 months on, 6 weeks off.

## VITAMIN C

The significance of vitamin C, also known as ascorbic acid, in maintaining homeostasis is truly fascinating. Although the human body cannot produce this essential nutrient, research has long shown the crucial role it plays in the protective effects of our immune system, especially because of its antioxidant effects.

Vitamin C is a critical cofactor for a range of essential enzymes and facilitates biochemical processes such as collagen synthesis. Vitamin C also acts as a cofactor in producing carnitine—the transporter that carries acids into mitochondria, the powerhouses of cells, where they are converted into the energy that drives all our actions. Vitamin C also supports the integrity of our autonomic nervous system and our fight-flight mode that protects our survival.

Vitamin C is a powerful anti-inflammatory agent that acts as an effective shield against reactive oxygen species (ROS) that can harm the body due to oxidative stress. The primary way in which vitamin C exerts its antioxidant power is by neutralizing free radicals—molecules that can cause damage to cells and tissues. Additionally, vitamin C inhibits enzymes responsible for generating ROS, effectively reducing their production at the root. This aspect is particularly important, since it implies that vitamin C not only cleans up after ROS but also prevents their formation in the first place.

Another crucial method through which vitamin C demonstrates its anti-inflammatory effects is by interacting with the NRF2 signaling pathway. By activating this pathway, vitamin C helps increase the production of antioxidant enzymes in cells, which enhances the cells' ability to fight against stress. Vitamin C plays a role in promoting cellular renewal, maintaining genetic integrity, and enhancing cell reprogramming, and it facilitates DNA demethylation, essential for preserving the vitality and function of stem cells.

Recent research has also pointed to vitamin C as playing a remarkable role in cancer biology, particularly in papillary thyroid carcinoma (PTC). Interestingly, the production of thyroid hormones is closely linked to hydrogen peroxide, and vitamin C influences this connection by regulating hydrogen peroxide levels within the thyroid.

## Dosage

First and foremost, it's important to understand that the levels of vitamin C in the blood are carefully regulated by the body. Vitamin C is indeed essential for our well-being; however, the body has mechanisms to maintain levels both in the bloodstream and within cells. The concentration of vitamin C in the blood is typically controlled within a range of 40 to 100 micromoles, which supports functions without exceeding optimal levels.

When vitamin C is taken orally, it is absorbed efficiently at intakes ranging from 30 to 180 mg daily. The absorption rates during this range are between 70% and 90%. However, when the dosage goes beyond 1 g daily, the efficiency of absorption decreases significantly and can be counterproductive. A closer examination of the pharmacokinetics reveals that an oral intake of 1.25 g daily leads to a peak concentration in the blood plasma of around 135 micromoles on average. This level is only slightly higher than what can be achieved with a dose of vitamin C–rich foods: approximately 200 to 300 mg daily. Interestingly, according to pharmacokinetic modeling predictions, even if you take an oral dose of ascorbic acid (vitamin C) every 4 hours totaling 3 g, it would only result in a peak plasma concentration of approximately 220 micromoles.

Taking high doses of vitamin C orally doesn't necessarily mean there will be significant improvement in the cells' redox state. Pursuing levels of antioxidants excessively can sometimes have negative effects, as the body has a regulated process for absorbing vitamin C. The cells themselves determine their requirements. There might be instances in which temporarily increasing the level of vitamin C in the blood to its maximum can be beneficial, such as during periods of stress or illness, when there is an increased demand for antioxidants. In these cases, having the ability to elevate blood levels through administration that bypasses absorption limitations could provide significant advantages. Vitamin C should be rotated 3 months on, 6 weeks off.

## VITAMINS D & K2

In this day and age, there is a prevailing deficiency in vitamin D that affects aspects of our well-being. This shortage sets the stage for diseases that can contribute to osteoporosis, different types of cancers, inflammatory bowel disease (IBD), mood and cognitive disorders, obesity, and a range of other diseases. However, amid this deficiency lies the biggest threat: a weakened immune system. As we face the challenges posed by viral and bacterial infections such as COVID-19, along with growing concern over antibiotic resistance, we must ask ourselves what can strengthen our defenses.

The answer lies in combining vitamin D with vitamin K2. When taken alone, vitamin D has the potential to lead to calcification, where excess calcium accumulates in areas, causing more harm than good. This is where vitamin K2 comes into play. When combined, the two vitamins set off a powerful chain reaction that not only prompts the body to produce more glutathione (GSH), a potent antioxidant, but also enhances its functionality. Vitamin K2 acts as a key to unlock vitamin D's potential by facilitating its activation. With levels of GSH, we witness our cells' mitochondria transform into resilient defenders of our immune system.

Vitamins D and K2 each possess strengths. Vitamin D stands tall as the guardian for bones—combating diseases, protecting immune defenses, positively influencing mood, and safeguarding against cardiovascular issues. Vitamin K2 serves as a carrier—ensuring that calcium reaches bones to fortify their strength, shielding the heart's arteries, silently fighting against cancer, enhancing insulin sensitivity, and providing relief from inflammation.

Vitamin D also boosts antioxidant enzymes and activates the NRF2 pathway, a mechanism for safeguarding our cells against stress. In addition, it regulates calcium signaling, an ally in combating oxygen species and thereby balancing redox.

## Dosage

My general recommendation is to take Vitamin D in the form of Vitamin D3 (cholescalciferol) for better absorption. While this supplement does not need to be rotated, blood levels should be noted regularly.

---

**NOTE** The Recommended Dietary Allowance (RDA) for vitamin D varies based on age: For infants, the RDA is 400 IU; for adults age 70 and over, the RDA is 800 IU or more. However, individuals who are deficient may need a higher dose to address their deficiency.

---

# The Three Pillars of **Cellular Resilience** and **Healthy Aging**



## PART 3

## HOW TO EAT FOR CELLULAR EFFICIENCY AND METABOLIC HEALTH

Of course we know the body needs food to grow and function. Of course we know some foods are good and some are not so good. But because we live in a world that is, let's just say, *enthusiastic* about food, and because processed foods are ubiquitous and pushed heavily by companies that know exactly how to trick our taste buds and create addictive-like dependencies on those hyper-palatable foods, it's super important to arm ourselves with accurate information about what to eat, when to eat, and how to eat.

What we eat sets the foundation for optimal cell metabolism; when we eat is crucial for enabling our cells to work efficiently; and how we eat (the order and combination of foods) sets us up to eat more of what we like without any of the negative side effects.

In other words, the what, when, and how of my approach to eating is about being flexible while trying your best to eat nutritiously most of the time. My approach is not restrictive, so those following the plan won't feel deprived or hungry, and it enables them to either lose weight or maintain their weight, depending on their goal.

When we consume nutrient-rich foods, we directly support the production and use of cellular energy and cellular efficiency. Foods that are processed, laden with fat and sugar, and otherwise devoid of nutrients that the body can break down and utilize short-circuit or undermine cellular metabolism and efficiency. These "bad" foods also upset the microbiome, cause inflammation, and can trigger a range of diseases from diabetes to obesity. At the same time, our body is meant to adapt, and enjoying a piece of cake or some fast food every once in a while challenges it to adapt. Don't get me wrong: I am not recommending fast food or sugary desserts; I am recommending changing up food choices so that the body is prompted to adapt and stay resilient.

My approach to eating is both simple and enjoyable. Two nutritional approaches that are supported by decades of scientific research are good starting points: the Mediterranean Diet and the Okinawa Diet. Both emphasize plant-based foods such as vegetables, fruits, legumes, and whole grains; deepwater fish; and a limited amount of protein from meat. The Okinawa diet in particular represents an approach to eating associated with *Blue Zones*, those areas in the world—Ikaria, Greece; Sardinia, Italy; Nicoya, Costa Rica; Okinawa, Japan; and Loma Linda, California—where people are known to live longer, healthier lives.

Both the Mediterranean and Okinawa diets also speak to an eating mindset: Eat to enjoy food, slow down, eat for pleasure, and gather together to eat and enjoy food with family or friends. And while neither approach restricts food based on calories, both tend to serve modest portions and avoid eating past fullness. This mindset not only allows the body to digest and absorb food better, it also encourages a healthy attitude toward food as nutrition.

I've also included some tips on how to incorporate intermittent fasting and how the timing of meals affects digestion and metabolism.

There's no one way to try fasting. In fact, it's not recommended for everyone. But there are some key ideas that will help us tweak our health goals.

The same goes for what we put on our plate and the order in which we eat certain foods. For example, if we start with proteins and save carbs for last, we will avoid the spike in blood sugar that often inhibits our satiety signal (the body's built-in signal that cues us to stop eating because we're satisfied/full).

People do best when they understand how nutritious food in moderate amounts will protect the brain, microbiome, and other cell systems. This way of eating is the essence of better aging—not only because it will make us look better and feel better (which it will), but also because it enables the cells of the body to work efficiently and fight disease, including those that affect the brain and memory.

## Food Basics

I like to keep things simple. While we live in a world of abundance, choosing good food is not always easy, especially if your budget is tight, you live far from stores that provide fresh food, or you are short on time. Another obstacle in the way of many well-intentioned eaters is the difficulty of sorting through all the seemingly contradictory information out there, including from Instagram, Facebook, and celebrity-sponsored eating plans: Avoid fat. Eat fat. Stay away from carbs. Pasta is good for you. Pasta is the devil . . . you get the picture. It's no wonder so many people are confused about how to even think about food!

Adding to the confusion are all the advertisements that try to reel us in with fast, cheap, and flavor-rich foods that we can eat anywhere and at any time. These foods are not only devoid of most nutrition, but also contain many chemicals that act like endocrine disrupters: powerful toxins that disrupt cellular metabolism and can also trigger disease.

Let me make one thing clear: I am not a purist when it comes to nutrition. I think of myself as more of a realist. I am not a vegetarian, though I do eat a lot of plant-based foods. I love to eat a burger and

French fries every once in a while. And though I don't drink alcohol, I do indulge in other pick-me-ups: I love coffee! We all have our go-to treats, and I think life would be boring without them. Given the shortness of life on this planet, you might as well enjoy food and drink . . . even if it's a bit "bad."

So, what I do to stay healthy is *stick to the basics*. I make sure I get a sufficient amount of clean protein with every meal. This might be one or two eggs in the morning, a serving of grilled chicken for lunch, and fish once or twice a week for dinner. I emphasize "clean" because you want your protein source to have as little "bad" fat as possible.

Which brings me to a key source of nutrition: fats. When it comes to protecting the brain, keeping the mind sharp, improving memory, ensuring a healthy microbiome, and reserving energy to prevent disease, fats are the answer.

The good news is that there are many delicious good fats—from olive oil, sunflower oil, and avocados to nuts and beans. Good sources of fat can be added to every meal.

## BAD FATS VERSUS GOOD FATS: UNDER THE MICROSCOPE

Under the microscope, so-called bad fats can be distinguished from good fats based on their makeup: Bad fats are even-chain saturated fatty acids and good fats are odd-chain saturated fatty acids (like pentadoceniac acid), monosaturated fats (olive oil), and polyunsaturated fats (omega-3 docosahexaenoic acid [DHA], eicosapentaenoic acid [EPA]).

Odd-chain fatty acids improve cardiac, metabolic, and anti-inflammatory health, whereas even-chain fatty acids are associated with negative health, increased coronary heart disease, increased bad cholesterol, type 2 diabetes, and pro-inflammatory states.

Good fats are essential for organ health, red blood cell health, strengthening the cell membranes, repairing mitochondria, and overall metabolism. Good fats are also essential for regulating appetite, mood, and sleep. Dietary odd-chain saturated fatty acids can lower risk of inflammation, type 2 diabetes, cardiometabolic disease, and both nonalcoholic fatty liver disease (NAFLD) and nonalcoholic steatohepatitis (NASH).

Of course, there are also plenty of bad fats, and it's often confusing to distinguish between what's good and what's bad. Here is my litmus test for knowing whether a fat is really bad for you:

- Fat attached to meat (e.g., chicken skin or marbled meat): It may taste good, but it's loaded with saturated fat that may be harmful. Higher intake means more potentially harmful effects. Bottom line: too much is too much, in both cases.

- Fat that comes with sugar (e.g., in ice cream, cakes, and cookies): Of course, there's always room to indulge in some deliciousness, but not every day, throughout the day. Also, it's important to note that most sugars that are not immediately used by the brain or body turn into fat, which is stored and deposited throughout the body in organs such as the liver as well as under the skin.

The third and possibly most important food on my plate is vegetables—the more colorful they are, the better. Remember, these are base foods that offset the acid-producing micronutrients. I include as many green vegetables as possible—salads, spinach, broccoli—along with colorful vegetables such as carrots, beets, peppers, and eggplant. These foods are high in many vitamins, minerals, and proteins that the body relies on to stay healthy. And though some starchy vegetables have a bad reputation for being highly glycemic and triggering cravings, I still enjoy potatoes, corn, and any vegetable from the squash family. Also, when paired with green vegetables and protein, starchy carbs will not trigger a spike in blood sugar or create cravings. Again, balancing protein and carbs is key to getting sufficient amounts of all that we need from foods without the negative side effects. In addition to vitamins and minerals, vegetables also provide insoluble fiber, which helps all the other food groups metabolize more easily. Fiber is also an important element to offset acid load and keep the microbiome balanced.

My approach works because it provides the brain and the body with the nutrition it needs to function optimally:

- Protein to build muscle, support tissues, and regulate the immune system (amino acid metabolism is key)

- Carbohydrates for energy (glucose metabolism is the brain and body's first source of fuel, and fiber helps balance the microbiome)

- Fats for healthy brain function and memory and to stabilize mood and fight against heart disease (fatty acids are the best source to fight effects of aging, including protecting the microbiome)

## WILLPOWER IS A MYTH

Hyper-palatable foods are addictive because they trigger a biochemical hit of pleasure (a surge of dopamine) that leaves us wanting more. This is the nature of any kind of craving, which can develop into a kind of addictive dependency, whether it's food, alcohol, or drugs. That's why quitting something "cold turkey" doesn't work. The patterns in our nervous system are super strong, making habits so hard to break. Our brain literally works against us.

But we do have some good options:

- We can discover new treats that will give our brain the "hit" it's looking for.

- We can work with the habit and outsmart it.

- We can time our treats so that they don't trigger a loss of control.

Again, The Redox Promise is not an all-or-nothing proposition. It's about balance, common sense, and listening to our body and our brain.

## Making Your Diet More Alkaline

Most of the processed foods in the Western (i.e., American) diet are highly acidic and cause the microbiome to go awry. Chronic acidity in the gut causes dysbiosis, inflammation, and a host of other diseases. A central way to restore the gut lining is to bring it back into pH balance.

This process doesn't happen overnight. We build acid load as we get older, which means the older we are, the more we need to pay attention to eating clean and balancing protein (acid producers) with bases (fruits and vegetables). Younger people get away with much more. In fact, young people can deal with excess protons/acidosis for a while before the acid buildup begins to wear on their microbiome. But those of us who are over the age of 40 need to pay attention to any signs of acidosis, including joint pain, dysbiosis, and inflammation. These are all signs that the microbiome is affected by a low-grade metabolic acidosis, and when that happens, it's a slippery slope that can lead not only to stubborn chronic conditions such as diabetes but also to Crohn's disease, irritable bowel syndrome (IBS), and even osteoarthritis.

I cannot emphasize enough the importance of maintaining pH balance based on dietary intake of proteins (acids) and fruits and vegetables (bases). It's possible to maintain pH balance by eating a clean diet that leans toward alkaline foods rather than those that create an acidic effect, but keep in mind the supplements described earlier that help with microbiome balance, including butyrate, bicarbonate (Alka Seltzer Gold), bovine colostrum, and lactulose.

**FOODS THAT PROMOTE ALKALINITY:**

Dark green vegetables

Citrus fruits

Pickles and cucumbers

Rice and other whole grains

Olive oil

Vinegar

**FOODS THAT HAVE AN ACIDIC EFFECT:**

Dairy

Pizza

French fries

Meat

Sweet sauces and condiments (ketchup, BBQ sauce, salad dressings)

Potato chips and other processed snacks

Alcohol

Desserts such as ice cream, cakes, and cookies

Note: you don't have to demonize dairy; dairy is a good source of pantadenoic acid and monosaturated fatty acid. The key is always to balance acid and alkaline foods.

---

## THE GOOD FOODS LIST

**FOODS THAT ARE GOOD FOR THE BRAIN (RICH SOURCE OF ODD-CHAIN SATURATED FATTY ACIDS)**

Avocados

Olive oil, sunflower oil

Nuts, especially walnuts and almonds

Note: walnuts are rich in alpha-linolenic acid, a plant-based omega-3; almonds have no omega-3s but do have other types of fatty acids.

**FOODS THAT ARE GOOD FOR THE GUT (FIBER + NATURAL PROBIOTICS)**

Green vegetables

Beans and legumes

Cabbage (including sauerkraut)

Pickles

Soy

Egg whites

Milk and dairy

It doesn't take a genius to recognize that some of our favorite "treats" have an acidic effect, which is why it's best to think of these as treats instead of everyday snacks. Also, the frying process makes otherwise nonacidic foods, such as potatoes, acidic. But because I am not a purist but a realist, it's not bad to indulge in any of these . . . in moderation. In fact, these hyper-palatable goodies can add a good kind of stress on our system, causing an adaptive response. Think of eating a bag of potato chips as a smoke detector going off, signaling that something foreign and potentially dangerous is in the house. The brain and body immediately detect the foreign invader (i.e., an unnatural food source) and gear up. The act of gearing up is the body's natural response to stress or toxins: The immune system is going to ramp up and attack.

However, if we eat potato chips every day, our body will adapt and the smoke alarm will no longer go off; as a result, our body will begin to absorb the fatty empty calories and store them as fat. The same is true for any of the foods on the acid hit list above.

### KEEP IN MIND

Most physicians consider a pH balance ranging from 7.35 to 7.45 to be normal.

## When to Eat

The timing of meals is important to both optimizing metabolism and maintaining a healthy weight. Although I recommend eating three meals a day, there are situations when two meals may be just as satisfying. And those who are trying out an intermittent fast may learn that eating one meal a day may work for them. However, as with anything, making radical changes too quickly can be detrimental. It's key to make one or two small adjustments at a time to monitor the effect of the change. Remember: We are our best guide as to what works . . . or doesn't work. The more attuned we are to our body, the more we will be able to make tweaks for better results.

**FIVE RULES FOR TIMING OF MEALS:**

- If considering intermittent fasting, delay breakfast to between 12 and 14 hours after the last meal the night before, ideally working up to 16 hours between meals.

- Don't snack in between meals unless you are exercising.

- Try to make dinner the smallest meal of the day and eat as early as possible in the evening to help your circadian rhythm.

- Avoid late-night meals or snacks.

- Finish eating at 6 p.m. so that you're ready to eat breakfast by 8 a.m.

## Fasting: How to Fast Safely and for Best Results

The science of fasting is clear: To fast in a way that optimizes metabolism, draws upon fat storage supplies, and increases energy, one must fast between 14 and 16 hours. That means if you eat dinner at 6 p.m. and eat nothing until the next day between 8 a.m. and 10 a.m., you will push your body and brain into a metabolic fasting state.

This may seem like too long a stretch to go without food. Again, it's not something I advise doing suddenly. You need to get your body (and your brain!) accustomed to this approach gradually. Perhaps start by going 12 hours—most people can eat a final meal at 7 p.m. and wait until 7 a.m. to have breakfast. And this 12-hour stretch is great for you anyway because it gives the body a necessary rest. Ideally, this rest is at night when the body is in rest-and-restore mode (see the section "How to Sleep to Support Your Immune System and Age Better" for more on the importance of rest and sleep for optimal metabolism).

Intermittent fasting is a type of calorie restriction, which in general I don't think is such a good idea on a daily basis. Why? Because I think it's simpler and more sustainable in the long run to try one or two days of intermittent fasting per week to prime the cellular metabolism to work more efficiently. Indeed, the research on calorie restriction (which was based on study participants eating two small meals daily) does show that its effect on metabolism and cell efficiency is similar to that of technical intermittent fasting. And again, both fasting and calorie restriction have been shown to make cells throughout the body function more efficiently. They've also been shown to reduce the risk of cancer. Unfortunately, a recent (2024) epidemiological study that demonizes intermittent fasting has scared people; this very narrow study stands in contrast to the plethora of scientific research that shows both the benefits and safety of fasting when done responsibly.

For me and my patients, fasting is the easier, more sustainable approach. With fasting, you can have water, tea, and black coffee, but no soda, juice, or other drinks with sugar or a sugar substitute. Any kind of sugar (i.e., carbohydrate) will turn off fat burning.

The difference between a fast that lasts for 10 to 12 hours and one that lasts for 14 to 16 hours is related to glucose metabolism. When the body goes without food for 14 to 16 hours, it moves into ketosis, so it burns fat to make ketones for energy. In the 10-to-12-hour fast, the blood glucose is not depleted enough, so the body does not go into ketosis.

However, it's still possible to burn fat without ketones . . . if you are also exercising. For instance, a long, low-intensity walk (20 to 30 minutes) tells the body that it has to sustain its energy, so it will begin to use fat! But a high-intensity session on a step machine uses glucose . . . you'd have to go for about an hour before your body uses fat. (See the following section on how best to integrate exercise into your routine for maximum cell efficiency and/or weight loss, if that's your goal!)

You can also fast every other day for 24 hours, which enables you to increase your metabolism and improve cell efficiency.

Another powerful way to regenerate the body and brain through fasting is to fast for 48 to 72 hours once every three months. This type of fast, which you should only consider doing under medical supervision, activates stem cells and changes the chemistry of the body through a prolonged state of ketosis. Again, I advise my patients to work up to this type of fast gradually, only after they are accustomed to intermittent fasting one or two days a week.

A good idea for the 48-to-72-hour fast would be to do it over a weekend, from a Friday through a Monday, when you are less likely to be working. This extended fast works like a detoxifying cleanse, replenishing your immune system, empowering cell efficiency, and heightening mental clarity. It's the ultimate brain boost.

## A NEW WAY TO LOOK AT FASTING AND TIME-RESTRICTED FEEDING

In my redox clinic, we've been developing a new approach to time-restricted feeding based on the latest research. Periodic restricted feeding for weight loss and improved metabolic health involves four days of restricted feeding and works like this:

1. Day 1: Eat 50% of what you normally eat.

2. Days 2, 3, and 4: Eat 35% of what you normally eat.

3. For the next 10 days, eat normally.

4. Begin the cycle again.

Many of my patients are enjoying significant results within 12 weeks and find they can sustain this cycle with ease. You can still achieve improved health and weight loss by cycling on and off. As I've recommended elsewhere, it's always beneficial to your health to eat a Mediterranean or Okinawa diet for best results.

## HOW TO EXERCISE TO IMPROVE STRENGTH, ENERGY, AND FOCUS

You've heard it before: Exercise is good for your health. Exercise is good for your heart. Exercise strengthens and tones your muscles. Exercise helps you lose weight and keeps you fit. It's all true . . . and yet, why is it so hard for many people to make exercise a regular part of their lives? Why do so many people promise themselves they will work out more, join a gym, and even pay for a trainer . . . and then a few weeks or months go by and they are back on the couch?

I think I have the answer: because many people do not fully appreciate the *why* of exercise. Exercise is literally—and I am not exaggerating—the magic bullet of wellness, especially as we age. Exercise not only keeps us fit on the outside, but it's also key to our *inside* fitness because it maximizes our cellular efficiency, which of course keeps us in the healthy aging zone. And as I've said, when cells function efficiently, they are more capable of keeping us in redox balance, supporting our immune system, and enabling us to maintain a high level of energy and focus. A sedentary lifestyle, one that does not include regular exercise, is basically an invitation for disease and a one-way ticket to bad aging.

The good news is that it's *never* too late to start an exercise regimen. Even better, my approach to exercise is similar to my approach to eating; that is, I'm not a purist, and I believe variety is best for the body and the brain and that all-or-nothing plans are not sustainable.

What follows is an approach you can take to make exercise a part of your life—on *almost* a daily basis. "Almost daily" doesn't mean it will take hours from your day or week. It also doesn't mean joining an expensive gym, buying a $2,000 bike, or signing up for a series of yoga or Pilates classes (although those might be good options if you have the resources).

The redox approach to exercise is far simpler, far more affordable, and far more doable. And it works. It will reinforce the dietary changes you are making so that you look and feel better. It will continue to prime your cell efficiency and, as a result, keep you healthy. It will give you more energy and redistribute weight from the hips and stomach to the legs. In other words, this approach is literally a no-brainer.

As you know, I rely on lots of scientific studies and a ton of research to back up any recommendation I make to my patients or my physician colleagues. Therefore, all the information and guidance in this section is backed by the latest in exercise science and substantive research, so you can count on it. Now you just have to do it!

## The Why of Exercise

A very simple definition of exercise is any activity requiring physical effort and carried out to sustain or improve health and fitness. At the cellular level, exercise is any movement that raises the heartbeat and circulates blood through the body, improving oxygenation of the cells, which means that exercise—its level of exertion and duration—varies according to who you are.

If you are a 90-year-old male who can no longer push a lawnmower, farm the fields, or play two sets of tennis, walking around the block is good exercise. Why? Because although the body is older and the cells are not as efficient as they were even 10 years ago, walking around the block still gets the heart pumping and the blood circulating, improving oxygenation of the cells. This is good for the brain, the muscles, the bones, and the joints . . . even if those joints ache a little more.

Why do I stress this example? Because it's a clear reminder that the simple actions we take every day can be good forms of exercise. Think gardening or cleaning the house. Or walking to and from the mailbox or up and down the stairs.

Obviously, exercise is also about exertion. When you walk around the block at a fast pace, you exert more energy. When you jog or run, either outside or on a treadmill, you increase your level of exertion. If you walk at a normal pace for about 45 minutes, even though you're not breathing heavily, your body will still use fat as its main source of fuel instead of relying on glucose. This means your body can burn fat more efficiently, which is good if you're trying to lose weight. It also improves the efficiency of adenosine triphosphate (ATP) production in the mitochondria, which is important for overall energy production in the body. When you lift weights, dance, or take a spin class, you raise your exertion level. But the fact remains that all of these forms of exercise are similar in that they raise the heart rate and circulate the blood, which helps the cells become more efficient.



## The What of Exercise

Although I stand by my simple definition of exercise, there are different forms of exercise that have different effects on the body. You've probably heard the terms *aerobic* and *anaerobic*. *Aerobic exercise* refers to any kind of movement that requires respiration—walking, running, dancing, skiing, and cycling are all forms of aerobic exercise. Aerobic conditioning requires oxygen and improves the body's ability to transport oxygen and clear out carbon dioxide. The more you train aerobically, the more you build your endurance.

*Anaerobic exercise* refers to any type of movement that does not utilize oxygen, and instead relies on the intensity of exertion. High Intensity Interval Training (HIIT), weight lifting, power yoga, CrossFit workouts, barre workouts, and Pilates are all forms of anaerobic exercise.

Anaerobic conditioning is when your body works out without oxygen, because of the intensity of the exertion. For example, walking at a swift pace will utilize oxygen to fuel the movement (and get the heart pumping and blood circulating). Running a 25-yard dash, however, is primarily anaerobic because the rate of exertion is more intense and there is little time to rely on oxygen to fuel the movement; instead, the movement comes from muscle exertion. It's for this reason that anaerobic activities help strengthen muscles and bones and improve cardiovascular endurance, which is so important to us as we age.

These terms can be helpful to keep in mind as you begin to figure out what exercise will most benefit *your* body. Again, variation is key to prompting your body (and your brain) to adapt. It's important that you switch up any exercise routine so that your muscles don't plateau.

I like to think about exercise as a natural extension of what you do every day. Think about what you do on a daily basis: carry a laundry basket, bend to pick up the newspaper, climb the stairs, or open the garage door. Think about the functions behind these motions. Carrying, pushing, and pulling require arm, back, and core strength. Bending requires flexibility. Climbing, walking, and running all require both aerobic and anaerobic conditioning. You get the picture. This is why activities such as gardening and cleaning the house can be forms of exercise. It's also why walking can be just as effective as running, especially if you're more likely to do it. And this is why it's important to pay attention to all the parts of your body, from the feet and legs to the core and upper body, as well as the arms and shoulders. It's also why good fitness is a balance of strength, flexibility, and cardio.

## The Importance of Exercise for Developing Strength

Developing strength becomes increasingly important as we age. With strength comes more muscle mass and less loss of muscle (sarcopenia).

Our muscles and bones need weight-bearing activities to keep them strong and supple. This does not mean you have to take up bench pressing. It means you have to become intentional about how to include weight-bearing activities into your workout routine. Did you know yoga and Pilates can be weight bearing? Yes, we can use our own body weight to create resistance against gravity. This is the principle behind pushups either on your knees or in a plank. However, walking, jogging, and using a stair climber or elliptical machine are also forms of weight-bearing exercises—but they don't represent true resistance training (see below for more on resistance training).

Another tip to keep in mind: Strengthening does not necessarily mean bulking up. Leave that to the gym rats and weight lifters. For most people, strengthening alerts your muscles and bones to turn on. Inside your body, your cellular redox responds to this call to action by improving utilization of glucose and increased oxidation. These activities turn on your body and work against the effects of aging, including senescence, as well as fight against both osteoporosis and sarcopenia. I believe out of all the exercise training, resistance training is most beneficial long term to maintain and preserve muscle as we age.

Resistance training improves and increases resting metabolism because of increased muscle mass and mitochondrial density. Muscle is more metabolically active then and requires more energy to maintain.

## The Importance of Exercise for Cellular Efficiency

In addition to improving glucose utilization and metabolic capacity in general, regular exercise also helps to regulate nutrient sensing pathways. Both insulin-like growth factor 1 (IGF-1) and IGF-1EC play important roles in muscle growth and repair in response to exercise-induced mechanical loading and muscle contraction. IGF-1 is acutely stimulated by mechanical contraction and promotes ribosomal biogenesis and translation, leading to the formation of new myofibril proteins. This ultimately contributes to muscle growth and repair. IGF-1EC (also known as mechano growth factor or MGF) is a splice variant of IGF-1 that is produced in response to mechanical loading and muscle damage. It is specifically important for satellite cell activation, promoting their proliferation and differentiation and leading to the formation of new muscle fibers and the repair of damaged muscle tissue. Together, the release of IGF-1 and IGF-1EC in response to mechanical loading and muscle contraction during exercise promotes muscle and cellular efficiencies, growth, and repair.

Satellite cells are a population of stem cells that are located on the surface of muscle fibers. They are activated in response to muscle damage, and they differentiate into new muscle cells to repair the damaged tissue. IGF-1EC promotes satellite cell activation by binding to its receptor on the surface of satellite cells, which activates a signaling pathway that leads to their proliferation and differentiation.

One of the unique features of IGF-1EC is that it has a long, unique C-terminal extension that is not present in other IGF-1 isoforms. This extension is responsible for the specific activation of satellite cells and its effects on muscle growth and repair. It has been shown to stimulate the expression of several genes that are involved in satellite cell proliferation and differentiation, including myoblast determination protein 1 and myogenin. In addition to promoting satellite cell activation, IGF-1EC also has other effects on muscle tissue. For example, it has been shown to stimulate the production of collagen, which is a structural protein that is important for muscle tissue integrity, and it has anti-apoptotic effects, meaning that it can protect muscle cells from cell death.

Overall, IGF-1EC is an important splice variant of IGF-1 that is specifically produced in response to mechanical loading and muscle damage. Its effects on satellite cell activation are crucial for maintaining muscle tissue integrity and promoting muscle growth and repair.

Another exercise-regulated nutrient sensing pathway is AMP-activated protein kinase (AMPK), which is activated in response to decreased intracellular ATP and changes in the ratio of nicotinamide adenine dinucleotide (NAD+) to reduced NAD+ (NADH). Its function is to preserve ATP by inhibiting both biosynthetic and anabolic pathways while simultaneously stimulating catabolic pathways to re-establish cellular energy stores. The increased concentration of $Ca^{2+}$ during muscle contraction can also directly activate AMPK and is implicated in the regulation of numerous intracellular proteins that mediate cellular transduction, including kinase C, calcineurin, and CaMKs. Both AMPK and CaMKII lead to activation of PGC-1alpha, a member of a family of transcriptional coactivators that regulate mitochondrial biogenesis.

Exercise can actually induce oxidative stress in a controlled manner, which triggers a cascade of cellular signaling pathways that regulate nutrient sensing. One such pathway is the mitogen-activated protein kinase (MAPK) cascade, which is a family of intracellular signaling molecules that includes ERK1/2, JNK, and p38. Activation of the MAPK cascade by exercise leads to the production of sestrins, which are proteins that play a role in regulating cellular metabolism and stress responses. Sestrins have been shown to activate the AMPK pathway, which regulates energy balance in cells.

Moreover, activation of the MAPK cascade inhibits the activity of mTOR complex 1 (mTORC1), a protein complex that plays a central role in regulating cellular growth and metabolism. By inhibiting mTORC1, exercise can stimulate autophagy, a process by which the cell degrades and recycles damaged proteins and organelles. (mTOR inhibition is a temporary process; later stages of muscle recovery require mTOR activation.)

Finally, exercise-induced activation of the MAPK cascade can also lead to the activation of PGC-1alpha, a transcriptional coactivator that plays a central role in regulating mitochondrial biogenesis and oxidative metabolism. Activation of PGC-1alpha increases the production of mitochondria in cells and improves the capacity of cells to generate energy from nutrients.

Overall, exercise-induced oxidative stress can regulate nutrient sensing by activating the MAPK cascade and producing sestrins, which in turn regulate cellular metabolism and stress responses. This can lead to improved energy balance, increased autophagy, and enhanced mitochondrial biogenesis and oxidative metabolism. Table 2 summarizes how exercise benefits various systems of the body.

**Table 2. Effects of Exercise on Human and Animal Models of Aging**

| VARIABLE (ORGAN OR SYSTEM) | OBSERVATION |
| --- | --- |
| Longevity and health span | • Decreased risk of death |
| Cardiopulmonary | • Improved maximal oxygen uptake ($\uparrow VO_2$ max)<br>• Improved atherosclerotic plaque composition (calcification only)<br>• Prevention of post–myocardial infarction complications<br>• Improved functional outcome in patients with heart failure with preserved ejection fraction<br>• Improved progenitor cell functional capacity<br>• Decreased endothelial oxidative stress, improved vascular endothelial function<br>• Increased hematopoietic stem cells |
| Muscle/bone/skin | • Prevention of age-associated muscle degeneration<br>• Reduced physical disability<br>• Reduced sarcopenia<br>• Improved muscle endurance<br>• Enhanced balance and motor coordination<br>• Improved skin structure<br>• Increased bone formation, decreased osteoporosis |
| Peripheral and central nervous systems | • Improved executive function and memory<br>• Prevention of Alzheimer's disease and other neurodegenerative diseases<br>• Improved neurogenesis, neurotrophins, growth factors, and synaptic markers<br>• Decreased inflammation<br>• Restoration of retinal ganglion cells<br>• Preservation of neuromuscular junctions<br>• Relaxation, decreased anxiety and depression |

| VARIABLE (ORGAN OR SYSTEM) | OBSERVATION |
| --- | --- |
| Metabolism and glucose control | • Decreased peripheral insulin resistance<br>• Decreased insulin secretion<br>• Increased glucagon, gluconeogenesis, and fatty acid metabolism<br>• Decreased A1c<br>• Increased insulin-independent glucose uptake |

## KEEP IN MIND: BONE LOSS

As we age, we tend to lose bone mass and density, which increases the risk of fractures and other bone-related injuries. This decline is particularly rapid in postmenopausal females due to hormonal changes. However, recent studies have shown that regular strengthening exercises such as weight lifting and resistance training can counteract this loss and weakening of bones. High-intensity resistance training has been found to be effective in increasing bone mineral density in postmenopausal females with osteopenia, a condition in which bone mineral density is lower than normal but not low enough to be classified as osteoporosis. Another study found that resistance training improved bone density and strength in older males and females. Additionally, regular strengthening exercises can improve muscle strength and coordination, which is important for preventing falls and other injuries, particularly in older adults who are at a higher risk of falls due to factors such as decreased muscle strength, poor balance, and reduced mobility. Overall, these studies suggest that regular strengthening exercises can stimulate the production of new bone tissue and improve muscle strength and coordination, helping to prevent falls and other injuries and counteracting the loss and weakening of bones that occurs with aging. We can detect osteoporosis and osteopenia using a bone density test. Also called a DEXA (dual energy x-ray absorptiometry) scan, the test measures bone strength. Doctors usually recommend weight-bearing exercise to strengthen bones.

- *Osteopenia* is when the bones lose some of their mineral content (especially calcium). With a lower mineral content, bones become weak, and the chance of a fracture increases.

- *Osteoporosis* is more severe and occurs when bones become more porous, making them likely to fracture easily. People with osteoporosis lose bone more quickly than they can grow new bone.

Keep in mind that people of any gender can develop osteoporosis, although it's more common in females. About 30% of postmenopausal females have osteoporosis.

Exercise is also about *duration*. Longer is not necessarily better. In other words, you don't have to be an ultramarathon runner to get good results. In fact, many marathoners, as well as many elite athletes, overtrain and begin to weaken their body. They overexert, carry too little body fat, and can often overstress the body to the point of injury, illness, or pure exhaustion.

It is possible for an athlete to look like they're in great shape but still be significantly overtraining and have impaired cellular redox. Overtraining is a condition that occurs when an athlete exceeds their body's ability to recover from exercise, leading to a prolonged period of fatigue, decreased performance, and increased risk of injury. One of the ways in which overtraining can lead to impaired cellular redox is through an increase in the production of reactive oxygen species (ROS). When the body is in a state of overtraining, ROS production can increase to the point where it overwhelms the body's antioxidant defenses, leading to oxidative stress. And as we know, oxidative stress can cause damage to cellular structures, including DNA, proteins, and lipids, which in turn impairs cellular redox, pushing the body down a slippery slope toward bad aging.

It is worth noting that overtraining can be difficult to detect, as it often presents with vague symptoms such as fatigue, decreased performance, and mood disturbances. Additionally, athletes who are overtraining may still appear to be in great physical shape, as their muscles may be hypertrophied and their body fat levels low.

To avoid overtraining and impairing cellular redox, athletes should follow a structured training program that includes appropriate periods of rest and recovery. Adequate nutrition and hydration is also important, as is paying attention to the warning signs of overtraining just mentioned. By taking a proactive approach to managing training load and recovery, athletes can maintain optimal cellular redox and prevent the negative effects of overtraining.

In fact, recent research has overwhelmingly concluded that the most impactful duration for exercise is quite short. In fact, a recent study published in 2021 showed that HIIT is more effective than moderate-intensity continuous training (MCT), which used to be considered the "gold standard."

So why do we exercise? To

- utilize more calories instead of storing them as fat,

- increase metabolic rate,

- sleep more soundly,

- lose inches,

- get rid of excess weight, and

- feel better.

All of these results happen when you make your cells more efficient through exercise. And it doesn't take a lot of exercise to get these results.

---

**KEEP IN MIND**

The magic of HIIT is its intensity and its short duration. Over time, HIIT will recondition the cells, making them more efficient. Specifically, if you do HIIT three or four times per week for at least 6 weeks, you will get the results you want—whether that is to lose pounds or inches, sleep more soundly, or have more energy during the day. And on the inside, your body will be using the calories from food more effectively.

Neopterin is a biomarker that has been suggested as a potential tool for detecting overtraining in athletes. Neopterin is a by-product of the immune system, produced and synthesized by activated macrophages in response to inflammation and oxidative stress. Activated macrophages are white blood cells that play a key role in the immune system's response to infection and injury.

The production of neopterin is closely linked to the activity of the immune system, as it is released by macrophages in response to cytokines, which are signaling molecules that are produced by immune cells in response to infection or injury. This means that neopterin levels can reflect the level of immune system activity in the body. It has been suggested that neopterin levels may increase in response to overtraining, due to the increased oxidative stress and inflammation associated with this condition. When an athlete exceeds their body's ability to recover from exercise, it can lead to a state of chronic inflammation and oxidative stress, which can impair immune function and lead to the production of cytokines and other inflammatory molecules.

Measuring neopterin levels can therefore provide insight into the level of immune system activity and inflammation in an athlete's body, and may be a useful tool for detecting overtraining. By monitoring neopterin levels over time, athletes and coaches can track changes in immune system activity and inflammation, and adjust training load and recovery accordingly to prevent the negative effects of overtraining.

Several studies have investigated the use of neopterin as a marker of overtraining in athletes. Overall, neopterin shows promise as a potential tool for detecting overtraining in athletes, but further research is needed to determine its accuracy and reliability in this context. In the meantime, athletes and coaches should continue to rely on a combination of subjective and objective measures to monitor training load and detect signs of overtraining, including changes in mood, fatigue, decreased performance, and increased injury risk.

The evidence suggests that aerobic capacity, often measured by $VO_2peak$, is the strongest predictor of future health and all-cause mortality. $VO_2peak$ represents the maximal amount of oxygen that a person can consume during exercise and is considered an important measure of cardiovascular fitness.

Several studies have shown that people with high cardiorespiratory fitness, as measured by $VO_2peak$, have a significantly lower risk of developing cardiovascular disease and premature mortality, even if they have established risk factors such as high body mass index, hypertension, or diabetes. This suggests that cardiorespiratory fitness is a powerful predictor of cardiovascular health and that improving cardiorespiratory fitness can have significant benefits for overall health and longevity.

HIIT has emerged as a popular and effective way to improve cardiorespiratory fitness in a time-efficient manner. HIIT involves short bursts of high-intensity exercise, alternated with periods of lower-intensity exercise or rest. Several studies have shown that HIIT can be as effective or more effective than traditional moderate-intensity continuous training for improving cardiorespiratory fitness, particularly in individuals with limited time to exercise.

## Making It Real: The How of Exercise

To truly make exercise part of a weekly routine (notice that I did not say "daily"; you can think of integrating exercise on a *weekly* basis), you do not need to do a HIIT workout more than three times a week; two to three times per week creates substantive changes to your body and your *inner fitness*, where the cellular redox is making positive shifts in both form and function.

It is important to set some goals for yourself. Goals help all of us organize our time and motivate us to stick to our routine. This does not mean you can't be flexible. If you wake up one morning and feel tired or achy, it's best to skip working out that day and get some rest instead. But in general, as you begin to identify the types of exercise you enjoy, mark down on your calendar when you plan to work out. Plan to walk with a friend or neighbor two or three times a week. If you prefer walking solo, fine. But most of us need to be intentional about both what we want to accomplish (i.e., our goals) and when, or else it doesn't happen.

It may seem like a cliché, but good goals are SMART goals. They are

*S*pecific: You have identified what type of exercise you want to try or do.

*M*easurable: You are able to track your progress by monitoring your results and outcomes.

*A*ttainable: You are realistically able to achieve your exercise goals.

*R*elevant: The goals are meaningful to you.

*T*ime bound: You've given yourself a reasonable amount of time to achieve the goals (over time).

When you use these criteria to guide your goal setting, you will both set yourself up for success and reinforce your motivation!

## Maintaining a Balance Between Working Hard and Hardly Working

The redox approach to exercise is all about balance and flexibility. You want to keep a balance between working hard and working too hard; that is, exercising two times a week for too long a duration. You also need to make sure you incorporate rest so that your body has a chance to restore and reset. This balance will improve your performance and your results.

It's also important to vary the types of exercise you do. This variability is about using the right amount of stress to alert your body. When you change your routine, even a little bit, it sets off an alarm for your body, telling it to pay attention and adapt.

In the end, my golden rule for exercise is simple: Do what you enjoy. Perhaps you make it social . . . or not. Perhaps you enjoy working out in the morning . . . or not. My point is, just do it when you can. And stay flexible and forgiving of yourself. Again, if you're too narrow or restrictive in your thinking, you will burn out.

## Aerobic Exercise for Cellular Efficiency and Redox Balance

*Walking Program*

This walking program focuses on fat utilization and avoids excessive reliance on glucose, and is therefore an effective approach for fat loss.

- Duration: 45 minutes

- Frequency: Daily (or at least 5 days a week)

- Warm-up: Start with a slow pace for 5 to 10 minutes to warm up the body and prepare for exercise.

- Main workout:

  - Duration: 35 to 40 minutes

  - Speed: Aim for a moderate pace of 2 to 4 mph (or about 3.2 to 6.4 km/h) on flat terrain.

  - Intensity: Keep your heart rate in the low to moderate range, around 60% to 70% of your maximum heart rate. You can use a heart rate monitor to help you stay within this range, or you can use a perceived exertion scale (aim for a 4 to 6 on a scale of 1 to 10).

  - Incline: If you are walking outdoors, you can incorporate some hills or inclines to add some variety and increase the intensity of the workout. Aim for a moderate incline of 3% to 5% for short periods of time.

  - Cool-down: End with a slow pace for 5 to 10 minutes to gradually lower your heart rate and prevent dizziness or fainting.

**TIPS FOR MAXIMIZING THE BENEFITS OF THIS PROGRAM:**

- Stay hydrated. Drink water before, during, and after the workout to help your body burn fat efficiently. (Sip on the Amino Drink all day!)

- Avoid high-carbohydrate meals or snacks before the workout. This can increase your reliance on glucose instead of fat as a fuel source.

- Consider fasting before the workout. If you are able to, exercising in a fasted state (without having eaten 12 to 16 hours before the workout) can help your body burn more fat during the workout.

- Incorporate strength training. Building lean muscle mass through strength training can increase your resting metabolic rate and help you burn more fat throughout the day, even when you are not exercising.

### *Aerobic Cycling Program*

Cycling is a good form of aerobic exercise. This program helps build endurance and supports heart health.

- Duration: 45 to 60 minutes

- Equipment needed: Stationary bike, water bottle, comfortable athletic clothing and shoes

- Warm-up: Start with 5 to 10 minutes of light pedaling to warm up the body and prepare for exercise.

- Main workout:

  - Increase resistance on the bike to a moderate level.

  - Alternate between 3 minutes of pedaling at a moderate pace and 1 minute of high-intensity pedaling.

  - Repeat this cycle for a total of 30 to 45 minutes.

  - Cool-down: End with 5 to 10 minutes of light pedaling to gradually lower your heart rate and prevent dizziness or fainting.

### TIPS FOR MAXIMIZING THE BENEFITS OF THIS PROGRAM:

- Start at a moderate pace and gradually increase the intensity and duration as your fitness level improves.

- Stay hydrated by drinking water throughout the workout. Remember: The Amino Drink can make workouts more metabolically efficient.

- Wear comfortable athletic clothing and shoes to prevent chafing or discomfort.

- Focus on maintaining good form throughout the workout to avoid injury and maximize muscle engagement.

- Incorporate other forms of cardio and resistance training to create a well-rounded fitness program.

- Always warm up and cool down properly to prevent injury and maximize the benefits of the workout.

- Make sure to give yourself at least one rest day between each workout session to allow for proper recovery.

The specific intensity and duration of the workout will depend on your fitness level and goals. It's important to consult with a certified personal trainer or exercise physiologist to determine the best cycling program for your individual needs.

### Aerobic HIIT Program

This simple step-up HIIT program can be accomplished in 7 minutes. The program consists of four intervals of the chosen exercise. After each 30-second burst is a 15-second rest period, and then immediately after that the 30-second exercise is repeated. This will happen four times.

There is also a 1-minute warm-up period and a 1-minute cool-down period.

Here is the step-by-step program:

1. Start with a light jog in place for 1 minute to warm up the body and prepare for exercise. This could also be a treadmill walk at 1.5 to 2.5 mph (2.4 to 3.2 km/h).

2. Choose from the following HIIT exercises to complete in four intervals of 30 seconds, with a 15-second rest between each:

   - Squat jumps: Perform deep squats followed by explosive jumps.

   - Burpees: From a standing position, move into a squat with your hands on the ground, then kick your legs out into a plank position. Do a push-up, pop back up into a squat, then jump up with your hands raised.

- Mountain climbers: From a plank position, rapidly alternate bringing your knees to your chest.

- High knees: Run in place, lifting your knees as high as possible.

- Jump rope: Jump over an imaginary or actual jump rope for intense cardio.

- Sprints: Run at maximum speed, either outdoors or on a treadmill.

- Jumping jacks: Jump with your legs spread wide and the hands overhead, then bring your legs together and your arms down to quickly elevate the heart rate.

- Speed skaters: Jump from side to side, bending your knees in a lunge position, and touch the floor with each leap.

- Plank jacks: From a plank position, jump your feet out and in rapidly.

- Push-up to side plank: Combine push-ups with alternating side planks.

- Lunge jumps: Alternate jumping lunges, switching legs mid-air.

- Kettlebell swings: Swing a kettlebell between your legs rapidly, keeping your hips back and your knees bent slightly.

- Box jumps: Jump on and off a sturdy elevated platform.

- Battle ropes: Intensely wave or slam a battle rope.

- Stair sprints: Run up a flight of stairs as quickly as possible.

- Step-ups: Find a sturdy elevated surface (6 to 12 inches) and step up onto it with one foot, then the other. In the opposite order, step down with one foot, then the other. Try to raise your knees high, exaggerating the stepping motion. Pump your arms to add momentum and intensity, or hold lightweight dumbbells to increase the difficulty of the exercise.

You can do the same exercise for each interval or change to a different one. The key is trying to keep the heart rate within 80% to 95% of the maximum rate during the interval. An easy way to calculate this is 220 − age = heart rate maximum.

3. After the last 15-second rest period, cool down by jogging lightly in place for 1 minute. You could also repeat the warm-up treadmill exercise or take a light bicycle spin.

**TIPS FOR MAXIMIZING THE BENEFITS OF THIS PROGRAM:**

- Do this program two or three times a week. You can do it before resistance training or as an off-day exercise.

- Do not do this program more than three times a week.

- On the days you don't do the HIIT program, I recommend a 45-minute walk.

- Focus on maintaining good form throughout each exercise to avoid injury and maximize muscle engagement.

## Resistance Exercise

Resistance exercise includes body weight, resistance band, weight machine, dumbbell or kettlebell, and free weight exercises (such as Olympic bar lifting).

*Anaerobic Bodyweight Program: Resistance Training*

This bodyweight program can be done three times a week and targets the entire body.

- Duration: 45 minutes
- Warm-up: Start with 5 to 10 minutes of light cardio to warm up the body and prepare for exercise.
- Circuit 1:
    - Push-ups: 3 sets, 10 to 15 reps per set
    - Bodyweight squats: 3 sets, 10 to 15 reps per set
    - Plank hold: 3 sets, 30 to 60 seconds per set

Rest for 1 to 2 minutes between each set.

- Circuit 2:
    - Walking lunges: 3 sets, 10 to 15 reps per leg, per set
    - Glute bridges: 3 sets, 10 to 15 reps
    - Superman hold: 3 sets, 30 to 60 seconds per set

Rest for 1 to 2 minutes between each set.

- Circuit 3:
    - Pull-ups or inverted rows: 3 sets, 10 to 15 reps per set
    - Mountain climbers: 3 sets, 30 to 60 seconds per set
    - Russian twists: 3 sets, 10 to 15 reps per side, per set

Rest for 1 to 2 minutes between each set.

- Cool-down: End with 5 to 10 minutes of light cardio and stretching to gradually lower your heart rate and prevent dizziness or fainting.

## TIPS FOR MAXIMIZING THE BENEFITS OF THIS PROGRAM:

- Focus on maintaining good form throughout each exercise to avoid injury and maximize muscle engagement.

- Gradually increase the intensity and duration of each exercise as your fitness level improves.

- Incorporate other forms of cardio and resistance training to create a well-rounded fitness program.

- Always warm up and cool down properly to prevent injury and maximize the benefits of the workout.

- Make sure to give yourself at least one rest day between each workout session to allow for proper recovery.

### Band Resistance Program

Resistance bands are a convenient and effective way to include strengthening exercises into your routine.

- Duration: 30 to 45 minutes

- Equipment needed: Resistance bands of varying resistance levels (light, medium, and heavy), a sturdy anchor point (such as a doorframe or a heavy piece of furniture), and a mat or towel for comfort

- Warm-up: Start with 5 to 10 minutes of light cardio to warm up the body and prepare for exercise.

- Circuit 1:

    - Banded push-ups: 3 sets, 10 to 15 reps per set

    - Banded squats: 3 sets, 10 to 15 reps per set

    - Banded rows: 3 sets, 10 to 15 reps per set

Rest for 1 to 2 minutes between each set.

- Circuit 2:

    - Banded lateral walks: 3 sets, 10 to 15 reps per side, per set

    - Banded glute bridges: 3 sets, 10 to 15 reps per side, per set

    - Banded pull-aparts: 3 sets, 10 to 15 reps per side, per set

Rest for 1 to 2 minutes between each set.

- Circuit 3:

    - Banded deadlifts: 3 sets, 10 to 15 reps per set

    - Banded shoulder presses: 3 sets, 10 to 15 reps per set

    - Banded leg curls: 3 sets, 10 to 15 reps per set

Rest for 1 to 2 minutes between each set.

- Cool-down: End with 5 to 10 minutes of light cardio and stretching to gradually lower your heart rate and prevent dizziness or fainting.

**TIPS FOR MAXIMIZING THE BENEFITS OF THIS PROGRAM:**

- Alternate the resistance level (light, medium, and heavy) to challenge your muscles and allow for progression as your fitness level improves.

- Use a sturdy anchor point to secure the resistance band in place, and make sure the band is securely fastened to avoid injury.

- Focus on maintaining good form throughout each exercise to avoid injury and maximize muscle engagement.

- Gradually increase the intensity and duration of each exercise as your fitness level improves.

- Incorporate other forms of cardio and resistance training to create a well-rounded fitness program.

- Always warm up and cool down properly to prevent injury and maximize the benefits of the workout.

- Make sure to give yourself at least one rest day between each workout session to allow for proper recovery.

Some recommended bands for resistance training include Thera-Band Resistance Bands, Fit Simplify Resistance Bands, and WODFitters Resistance Bands. Choose the resistance level based on your fitness level and the exercises you will be doing.

*Circuit-Based Resistance Training Program*

Dumbbells are a classic method of strengthening the arms and shoulders.

- Duration: 30 to 45 minutes

- Equipment needed: Dumbbells of varying weights (light, medium, and heavy), a bench or stable surface, and a mat or towel for comfort

- Warm-up: Start with 5 to 10 minutes of light cardio to warm up the body and prepare for exercise.

- Circuit 1:

  - Goblet squats: 3 sets, 12 to 15 reps

  - Bench press: 3 sets, 12 to 15 reps

  - Bent-over rows: 3 sets, 12 to 15 reps

  - Plank: Hold for 30 seconds

Perform each exercise one after the other with no rest in between. After completing all four exercises, rest for 1 to 2 minutes and repeat the circuit for a total of three sets.

- Circuit 2:
    - Lunges with dumbbells: 3 sets, 12 to 15 reps per leg
    - Seated shoulder press: 3 sets, 12 to 15 reps
    - Bicep curls: 3 sets, 12 to 15 reps
    - Side plank: Hold for 30 seconds per side

Perform each exercise one after the other with no rest in between. After completing all four exercises, rest for 1 to 2 minutes and repeat the circuit for a total of three sets.

- Circuit 3:
    - Romanian deadlifts: 3 sets, 12 to 15 reps
    - Triceps extensions: 3 sets, 12 to 15 reps
    - Lateral raises: 3 sets, 12 to 15 reps
    - Bicycle crunches: 20 reps

Perform each exercise one after the other with no rest in between. After completing all four exercises, rest for 1 to 2 minutes and repeat the circuit for a total of three sets.

- Cool-down: End with 5 to 10 minutes of light cardio and stretching to gradually lower your heart rate and prevent dizziness or fainting.

**TIPS FOR MAXIMIZING THE BENEFITS OF THIS PROGRAM:**

- Choose dumbbells of varying weights (light, medium, and heavy) to challenge your muscles and allow for progression as your fitness level improves.

- Focus on maintaining good form throughout each exercise to avoid injury and maximize muscle engagement.

- Gradually increase the intensity and duration of each exercise as your fitness level improves.

- Incorporate other forms of cardio and resistance training to create a well-rounded fitness program.

- Always warm up and cool down properly to prevent injury and maximize the benefits of the workout.

- Make sure to give yourself at least one rest day between each workout session to allow for proper recovery.

The number of reps and sets and the weight of the dumbbells you use will depend on your fitness level and goals. It's important to consult with a certified personal trainer or exercise physiologist to determine the best resistance training program for your individual needs.

*Machine-Based Weight Lifting Program*

This machine-based weight-lifting program targets a variety of different muscle groups.

A: Consider a whole-body workout, three times a week, with a rest day in between.

B: Pick a body part, choose three machines to work it out, and do 2 or 3 sets, 10 to 12 reps (four days per week).

- Duration: 45 to 60 minutes

- Equipment needed: Weight-lifting machines (e.g., leg press, chest press, lat pulldown), water bottle, comfortable athletic clothing and shoes

- Warm-up: Start with 5 to 10 minutes of light cardio to warm up the body and prepare for exercise.

- Main workout:

  - Choose 8 to 10 weight-lifting machines that target different muscle groups, such as legs, chest, back, shoulders, and arms.

  - Perform 2 or 3 sets of 10 to 12 repetitions on each machine.

- Choose a weight that allows you to complete the repetitions with good form but still challenges you.

  - Rest for 30 to 60 seconds between each set.

  - Finish each set with a controlled eccentric (negative) phase of the movement to maximize muscle engagement.

- Cool-down: End with 5 to 10 minutes of light cardio and stretching to gradually lower your heart rate and prevent dizziness or fainting.

**TIPS FOR MAXIMIZING THE BENEFITS OF THIS PROGRAM:**

- Start with a weight that allows you to complete the repetitions with good form but still challenges you, and gradually increase the weight as your fitness level improves.

- Focus on maintaining good form throughout each exercise to avoid injury and maximize muscle engagement.

- Incorporate other forms of cardio and resistance training to create a well-rounded fitness program.

- Always warm up and cool down properly to prevent injury and maximize the benefits of the workout.

- Make sure to give yourself at least one rest day between each workout session to allow for proper recovery.

The specific weight, number of repetitions, and sets you incorporate into your program will depend on your fitness level and goals. It's important to consult with a certified personal trainer or exercise physiologist to determine the best weight-lifting program for your individual needs.

*Free Weights*

This resistance program uses free weights and focuses on strength improvement and muscle growth.

This is a well-rounded, weekly free-weight program that incorporates compound movements and exercises to target all major muscle groups. As a three-day program, it allows sufficient time for repair and recovery. Follow this schedule for 12 weeks, and then you'll be ready to explore other routines. Focus on one body part each day and consider taking the weekend off or enjoying light cardio on those days.

If you wish to take it one step further, consider combining HIIT and resistance training for two days out of the week, performing the HIIT routine before the resistance training. This has two major potential benefits:

- Enhanced warm-up: Performing HIIT before resistance training can serve as an effective warm-up, increasing blood flow and muscle temperature, which may enhance performance during subsequent resistance exercises.

- Increased metabolic stress: The metabolic stress induced by HIIT could potentially prime the muscles for greater adaptations during resistance training.

### MONDAY: LOWER BODY FOCUS

1. Barbell back squat: 4 sets, 6 to 8 reps

2. Romanian deadlift: 3 sets, 8 to 10 reps

3. Walking lunges with dumbbells: 3 sets, 10 to 12 reps per leg

4. Standing calf raises: 3 sets, 12 to 15 reps

5. Plank: 3 sets, 30 to 60 seconds

### WEDNESDAY: UPPER BODY FOCUS

1. Barbell bench press: 4 sets, 6 to 8 reps

2. Overhead press: 3 sets, 8 to 10 reps

3. Incline dumbbell press: 3 sets, 10 to 12 reps

4. Triceps dips: 3 sets, 10 to 12 reps

5. Lateral raises: 3 sets, 12 to 15 reps

### FRIDAY: BACK AND BICEPS FOCUS

1. Conventional deadlift: 4 sets, 6 to 8 reps

2. Bent-over barbell rows: 3 sets, 8 to 10 reps

3. Pull-ups or lat pull-downs: 3 sets, 8 to 10 reps

4. One-arm dumbbell rows: 3 sets, 10 to 12 reps per arm

5. Barbell or dumbbell bicep curls: 3 sets, 10 to 12 reps

This program hits all major muscle groups over the course of the week:

- Legs: Squats, lunges, calf raises
- Chest: Bench presses, incline presses
- Back: Deadlifts, rows, pull-ups
- Shoulders: Overhead presses, lateral raises
- Arms: Bicep curls, triceps dips
- Core: Planks and engagement during compound lifts

**TIPS FOR MAXIMIZING THE BENEFITS OF THIS PROGRAM:**

- Start each workout with a compound movement (e.g., squat, bench press, deadlift).
- Incorporate both pushing and pulling movements.
- Include exercises for larger and smaller muscle groups
- Allow at least one day of rest between workouts.
- Adjust weights, sets, and reps based on your fitness level and goals.
- Always use proper form and warm up before lifting.
- Start with weights you can handle safely and progressively increase the load as you get stronger. Include proper warm-up, cool-down, and stretching in your routine.

To seriously work on strength gains, follow this recommended weight progression for the bigger compound movements:

- Week 1: 50% of 1RM (one repetition maximum)
- Week 2: 60% of 1RM

- Week 3: 70% of 1RM

- Week 4: 80% of 1RM

- Week 5: 85% of 1RM

The specific weight, number of repetitions, and sets you incorporate into your program will depend on your fitness level and goals. Consult with a certified personal trainer or exercise physiologist to determine the best weight-lifting program for your individual needs.

## The Power of Visualization

Using the power of visualization has a tremendous effect on any activity—physical or mental—that we engage in. I learned this technique through weight training, but I apply it to everything I do. Indeed, visualization is a technique used by many athletes to improve their performance and enhance their mind–body connection during exercise. Essentially, visualization involves mentally rehearsing or "seeing" yourself performing an exercise or physical activity in a positive and successful way.

Research has shown that visualization can have a positive impact on physical performance, such as improving muscle strength, endurance, and accuracy, as well as reducing anxiety and increasing confidence in athletes. Visualization can also improve the mind–body connection, allowing individuals to better connect with their body and improve their overall physical and mental well-being.

One possible reason why visualization is effective is because it activates the same neural pathways in the brain that are involved in actual physical movement. By mentally rehearsing an exercise, individuals can strengthen the neural connections between their brain and muscles, improving their ability to perform the exercise with greater ease and efficiency.

Additionally, visualization can help to reduce anxiety and increase confidence by allowing individuals to mentally prepare for an upcoming exercise or activity. This can help to alleviate any fears or doubts they may have and increase their overall sense of readiness and focus.

To incorporate visualization into your exercise routine, try taking a few minutes before your workout to mentally rehearse each exercise, visualizing yourself performing each movement with precision, ease, and success. You can also use positive self-talk and affirmations to reinforce your visualization and build confidence in your abilities.

Overall, visualization can be a powerful tool for improving physical performance and enhancing the mind–body connection during exercise.

## HOW TO SLEEP TO SUPPORT YOUR IMMUNE SYSTEM AND AGE BETTER

Sleep. You yearn for it. You worry about it. You fear you're not getting enough of it. You love it, and sometimes you hate that you need it. Why all of these mixed emotions about sleep?

In some ways, sleep is very simple in its purpose: It enables the brain and body to rest and restore so that we feel more refreshed and energetic the next day. This may seem simple—we need sleep to rest up for the next day—but sleep does much, much more than that. It allows for a complicated set of processes that allow the body and brain to restore homeostasis, fight inflammation at the heart of bad aging, and re-energize functioning at the cellular level. Which is why it's so troubling to me that for many people, sleep—especially high-quality, restorative sleep—is difficult to achieve. Indeed, recent studies indicate that almost 2 billion people worldwide suffer from some sort of sleep disorder, including sleep apnea and/or insomnia. And sadly, most of these 2 billion people go undiagnosed and therefore untreated.

How well we sleep—in terms of both duration *and* quality—plays a vital role in how well our brain and body can stay healthy. Sleep enables the brain to clear out toxins that build up during the day; reset hormone and other neurochemical levels; consolidate memories important for learning and other cognitive functions; and protect against illness and disease. Sleep is also paramount for maintaining stable moods and emotional regulation.

At a cellular level, all of these physiological activities enable the brain and body to maintain overall homeostasis. In this way, sleep is a regulatory process. But to truly appreciate how to maximize sleep quality so that you give your brain and body enough time to rest, reset, and restore itself, you also have to keep in mind that sleep is complicated. It involves two underlying biological processes: our sleep drive, the physical need for sleep that's as strong and necessary as the drive to eat; and our inner clock that cues us to go to sleep, which we refer to as the *circadian clock*. These two distinct but interrelated processes work in tandem so that we go to sleep, stay asleep, and wake up feeling refreshed. However, as mentioned above, a lot of people experience difficulty in one or more ways. For example, they have trouble falling asleep, have trouble staying asleep, dream excessively, or move during their sleep. Any one of these can disrupt sleep quality, which in turn affects how well the brain and body reset during the night.

The irony, however, is that although we are learning more about how important sleep is to our quality of life both every day and over the course of our lives, sleep remains somewhat mysterious. As Johns Hopkins sleep expert Mark Wu, MD, PhD, points out: "Sleep is the only essential behavior whose function remains unknown. In addition, the molecular and cellular mechanisms regulating sleep remain poorly understood."

This section is intended to help clarify misunderstandings and offer clear, accurate information about what we *do* know about sleep and what we can do about it. In society today, being exposed to artificial light, technological noise, and distractions and traveling through different time zones have become somewhat normal and expected, but not enough attention has been paid to their deleterious effects on how they disrupt our ability to sleep well.

## Sleep Basics

In general, sleep is either light or deep and is either REM or non-REM, the latter which refers to whether sleep includes dreams or not. We cycle through four stages or states of sleep, with each stage presenting its own brain wave (as measured by an EEG) that reflects how much or how little brain activity is happening within that stage.

Stage 1, which is relatively short, occurs when you first fall asleep; your heartbeat and breathing slow down and your muscles relax. Stage 2 is the longest part of the sleep cycle; it's characterized by light sleep, a drop in body temperature, cessation of eye movements, and a slowing down of brain wave activity. Stage 3 is a period of deep sleep and happens in the first half of the night; this is the type of sleep that's most acutely tied to the feeling we have of waking up refreshed.

Both stage 3 and stage 4 sleep (also known as slow-wave sleep or SWS) are important for physical and mental health, and they serve different functions. During stage 3 sleep, the body undergoes physical restoration and repair, such as muscle growth and tissue repair. This stage is also important for strengthening the immune system, which helps protect the body against infections and diseases. During stage 4 sleep, the brain processes and consolidates memories, which is important for learning and retaining information. It is also during this stage that the brain flushes out metabolic waste products that build up during waking hours, which may help prevent neurological disorders; this process is known as *glymphatic drainage*.

Overall, both stage 3 and stage 4 sleep are important for maintaining optimal health and well-being, and it is essential to get enough of both stages of sleep for overall health. The ideal proportion of stage 3 and stage 4 sleep varies from person to person and can change throughout the lifespan, but a healthy adult typically spends about 20% to 25% of their sleep time in SWS (combining stages 3 and 4) and about 20% to 25% of their sleep time in REM sleep. In REM sleep, the brain is most active (i.e., dreaming). Interestingly, during this period, your heart rate and blood pressure resemble your typical daytime levels.

## SLEEP IS ESSENTIAL AND SERVES MULTIPLE PURPOSES

Most researchers agree that sleep regulation does not have one particular physiological purpose, but rather is essential for many purposes, including the following:

- development
- energy conservation/brain waste clearing
- modulation of immune response

- cognition

- performance

- vigilance

- disease

- psychological states

Again, sleep plays a critical role in maintaining redox balance, which is the balance between oxidants and antioxidants in the body. One way that sleep improves redox is by increasing the production of nicotinamide adenine dinucleotide phosphate (NADPH), which is an important reducing agent that helps neutralize oxidants and maintain redox balance.

Research has shown that NADPH production is highest during the night, when we are asleep. This is because the enzymes involved in NADPH production are regulated by the circadian clock, which controls many physiological processes in the body, including sleep–wake cycles.

During sleep, the body's metabolic rate decreases, and energy is redirected toward repairing and rejuvenating processes. This allows for an increase in NADPH production, which helps to counteract the effects of oxidative stress that can accumulate during the day.

NADPH is also important for other processes in the body, such as the synthesis of fatty acids and the regeneration of antioxidants such as glutathione (GSH). By increasing NADPH production at night, sleep helps to maintain a healthy redox balance, which is important for general health and well-being. Overall, the relationship between sleep and redox is complex, and there are many factors that influence this balance. However, it is clear that sleep plays a critical role in maintaining redox balance, and by increasing NADPH production at night, sleep helps to counteract the effects of oxidative stress and promotes optimal health.

## Sleep Recommendations

Not surprisingly, the quality and duration of sleep affect redox balance. The good news is that a lot of research is being conducted in this field, and we are learning more and more about how sleep works and why it's so important. For now, I want to leave with you some basic but powerful guidelines that your patients can use for creating healthy sleep habits and achieving sufficient high-quality sleep.

- Go to bed at around the same time each night. Current research says that the sweet spot is between 10 p.m. and 11 p.m.

- Wake up at around the same time each morning so that you approximate between 7 and 8 hours of sleep each night.

- Stop eating and drinking at least three hours before going to bed; this includes alcohol. And remember, alcohol will wake you up in the middle of the night when your body tries to metabolize it.

- Keep caffeine consumption to the early part of the day, avoiding it after 3 p.m. or so. Note that some people are more sensitive to caffeine than others. For instance, I can keep drinking coffee until 6 p.m. when I am working long days (and nights!), and it does not interfere with my falling asleep or staying asleep. But for some, a cup of tea or coffee after 2 p.m. can interfere with their sleep.

- Be conscious of the timing of your exercise. Again, this varies. Many people find that exercising later in the day is relaxing, and others find it too stimulating. You be the judge.

- In extreme cases of sleep dysregulation, some of my patients have benefitted from CBD creams or tinctures.

- Melatonin (3 to 10 mg) can help people fall asleep.

- Consider mouth taping for sleep apnea.

In extreme cases of sleep dysregulation, electromagnetic interventions such as pulsed electromagnetic field (PEMF) therapy (which is based on NASA technology) can regulate the interaction between the sleep drive and circadian rhythm. This technology can literally put you into stage 4 sleep. I have had great success with this type of intervention. Though still an emerging field, preliminary studies suggest PEMF exposure may positively impact sleep through its effects on melatonin and mitochondrial function. Specifically, small trials show PEMF applied before bedtime can increase endogenous melatonin levels, which regulates circadian rhythms. Animal research also indicates PEMF may enhance mitochondrial adenosine triphosphate (ATP) production and membrane potential, improving cellular bioenergetics that influence sleep cycles. Thus, PEMF may modulate hormones and optimize energy pathways involved in sleep regulation. However, current evidence has limitations including small sample sizes and lack of controlled trials in humans. High-quality randomized studies are still needed to establish clear efficacy, optimal treatment parameters, and underlying mechanisms of how PEMF may improve sleep. But the initial findings are promising. With further rigorous research, PEMF could emerge as an innovative, nonpharmacological approach to manage sleep disorders and improve sleep quality through effects on melatonin signaling, mitochondrial function optimization, and other cellular processes. The potential of PEMF warrants continued investigation in this area.

A final recommendation: Try napping. Studies have shown that taking a nap during the day can lead to improvements in glucose metabolism and insulin sensitivity, both of which are important for maintaining overall metabolic health. For example, a study published in *Diabetes Care* found that taking a 30-minute nap after lunch improved glucose metabolism in healthy adults. Another study, published in the *Journal of Clinical Endocrinology and Metabolism*, found that taking a nap during the day improved insulin sensitivity in healthy individuals. In addition, a study published in *Sleep Medicine* found that taking a 30-minute nap during the day led to changes in the expression of genes involved in metabolism and energy regulation. And a study published in *Neurobiology of Aging* found that taking a 1-hour nap in the afternoon was associated with better cognitive performance in older adults.

Overall, while the precise mechanisms by which napping affects cell metabolism are not fully understood, there is growing evidence to suggest that napping can have important effects on metabolic health.

## CLOSING THOUGHTS

It has become my life's mission to educate not only physicians and other healthcare practitioners but also my patients. I hope that with this book I have conveyed the importance of redox balance to overall health and its potential to age better so that all readers feel motivated to be proactive in protecting their cellular health. Today we have the power to understand how diseases blamed on aging can be avoided. We also have the power to apply and utilize the science of cellular medicine to unlock the secrets of how to age better so that we do not simply extend our lifespan but improve our *health span*.

Please feel free to reach out to our growing community of cellular medicine experts at the SSRP Institute. To find out more about how you can get involved, contact info@ssrpinstitute.org or visit the SSRP website, www.ssrpinstitute.org. And of course, you're welcome to follow me on Instagram @williamaseedsmd.

# BIBLIOGRAPHY


## REDOX

Birben, E., Sahiner, U. M., Sackesen, C., Erzurum, S., & Kalayci, O. (2012). Oxidative stress and antioxidant defense. *World Allergy Organization Journal*, 5, 9–19. http://doi.org/10.1097/WOX.0b013e3182439613

Gerwyn, M., Gevezova, M., Sarafian, V., & Maes, M. (2022). Redox regulation of the immune response. *Cellular & Molecular Immunology*, 19(10), 1079–1101. https://doi.org/10.1038/s41423-022-00902-0

Jones, R. M., & Neish, A. S. (2013). Redox signaling mediated by the gut microbiota. *Free Radical Research*, 47(11), 950–957. https://doi.org/10.3109/1071576 2.2013.833331

Kunst, C., Schmid, S., Michalski, M., Tümen, D., Buttenschön, J., Müller, M., & Gülow, K. (2023). The influence of gut microbiota on oxidative stress and the immune system. *Biomedicines*, 11(5), 1388. http://doi.org/10.3390 /biomedicines11051388

Le Gal, K., Schmidt, E. E., & Sayin, V. I. (2021). Cellular redox homeostasis. *Antioxidants*, 10(9), 1377. https://doi.org/10.3390/antiox10091377

Sies, H. (2015). Oxidative stress: A concept in redox biology and medicine. *Redox Biology*, 4, 180–183. http://doi.org/10.1016/j.redox.2015.01.002

Singh, C. K., Chhabra, G., Ndiaye, M. A., Garcia-Peterson, L. M., Mack, N. J., & Ahmad, N. (2018). The role of sirtuins in antioxidant and redox signaling. *Antioxidant Redox Signaling*, 28(8), 643–661. http://doi.org/10.1089 /ars.2017.7290

Trachootham, D., Lu, W., Ogasawara, M. A., Nilsa, R. D., & Huang, P. (2008). Redox regulation of cell survival. *Antioxidant Redox Signaling*, 10(8), 1343–1374. http://doi.org/10.1089/ars.2007.1957

Tretter, V., Hochreiter, B., Zach, M. L., Krenn, K., & Ulrich Klein, K. (2021). Understanding cellular redox homeostasis: A challenge for precision medicine.

*International Journal of Molecular Sciences*, 23(1), 106. https://doi.org/10.3390
/ijms23010106

Vardar Acar, N., & Köksal Özgül, R. (2023). The bridge between cell survival and
cell death: Reactive oxygen species-mediated cellular stress. *EXCLI Journal*,
22, 520–555. https://doi.org/10.17179/excli2023-6221

Willems, P. H., Rossignol, R., Dieteren, C. E., Murphy, M. P., & Koopman, W. J.
(2015). Redox homeostasis and mitochondrial dynamics. *Cell Metabolism*,
22(2), 207–218. http://doi.org/10.1016/j.cmet.2015.06.006

Xiong, Y., Uys, J. D., Tew, K. D., & Townsend, D. M. (2011). S-glutathionylation:
From molecular mechanisms to health outcomes. *Antioxidants & Redox Signaling*, 15(1), 233–270. https://doi.org/10.1089/ars.2010.3540

Zuo, J., Zhang, Z., Luo, M., Zhou, L., Nice, E. C., Zhang, W., Wang, C., &
Huang, C. (2022). Redox signaling at the crossroads of human health and disease. *MedComm*, 3(2), e127. http://doi.org/10.1002/mco2.127


## MICROBIOME

Aviello, G., & Knaus, U. G. (2018). NADPH oxidases and ROS signaling in the
gastrointestinal tract. *Mucosal Immunology*, 11, 1011–1023. http://doi
.org/10.1038/s41385-018-0021-8

De Vos, W. M., Tilg, H., van Hul, M., & Cani, P. D. (2022). Gut microbiome and
health: Mechanistic insights. *Gut*, 71, 1020–1032. http://doi.org/10.1136/
gutjnl-2021-326789

Hrncir, T., Hrncirova, L., Kverka, M., Hromadka, R., Machova, V., Trckova, E.,
Kostovcikova, K., Kralickova, P., Krejsek, J., & Tlaskalova-Hogenova, H.
(2021). Gut microbiota and NAFLD: Pathogenetic mechanisms, microbiota
signatures, and therapeutic interventions. *Microorganisms*, 9, 957. http://doi
.org/10.3390/microorganisms9050957

Kunst, C., Schmid, S., Michalski, M., Tümen, D., Buttenschön, J., Müller, M.,
& Gülow, K. (2023). The influence of gut microbiota on oxidative stress
and the immune system. *Biomedicines*, 11(5), 1388. http://doi.org/0.3390
/biomedicines11051388

Neish, A. S. (2013). Redox signaling mediated by the gut microbiota. *Free Radical
Research*, 47, 950–957. http://doi.org/10.3109/10715762.2013.833331

Shandilya, S., Kumar, S., Kumar Jha, N., Kumar Kesari, K., & Ruokolainen, J.
(2022). Interplay of gut microbiota and oxidative stress: Perspective on neurodegeneration and neuroprotection. *Journal of Advanced Research*, 38, 223–244.
http://doi.org/10.1016/j.jare.2021.09.005

Silva, Y. P., Bernardi, A., & Frozza, R. L. (2020). The role of short-chain fatty acids from gut microbiota in gut-brain communication. *Frontiers in Endocrinology*, 11, 25. http://doi.org/10.3389/fendo.2020.00025

Singh, V., Ahlawat, S., Mohan, H., Gill, S. S., & Sharma, K. K. (2022). Balancing reactive oxygen species generation by rebooting gut microbiota. *Journal of Applied Microbiology*, 132, 4112–4129. http://doi.org/10.1111/jam.15504

Wang, Y., Wu, Y., Wang, Y., Xu, H., Mei, X., Yu, D., Wang, Y., & Li, W. (2017). Antioxidant properties of probiotic bacteria. *Nutrients*, 9, 521. http://doi.org/10.3390/nu9050521

Wang, Y., Zhang, Z., Li, B., He, B., Li, L., Nice, E. C., Zhang, W., & Xu, J. (2022). New insights into the gut microbiota in neurodegenerative diseases from the perspective of redox homeostasis. *Antioxidants*, 11, 2287. http://doi.org/10.3390/antiox11112287

## CALORIE RESTRICTION

Charlot, A., Hutt, F., Sabatier, E., & Zoll, J. (2021). Beneficial effects of early time-restricted feeding on metabolic diseases: Importance of aligning food habits with the circadian clock. *Nutrients*, 13, 1405. https://doi.org/10.3390/nu13051405

Hoddy, K. K., Marlatt, K. L., Çetinkaya, H., & Ravussin, E. (2020). Intermittent fasting and metabolic health: From religious fast to time-restricted feeding. *Obesity*, 28, S29–S37. https://doi.org/10.1002/oby.22829

Li, M. D. (2022). Clock-modulated checkpoints in time-restricted eating. *Trends in Molecular Medicine*, 28, 25–35. https://doi.org/10.1016/j.molmed.2021.10.006

Patterson, R. E., & Sears, D. D. (2017). Metabolic effects of intermittent fasting. *Annual Review of Nutrition*, 37, 371–393. https://doi.org/10.1146/annurev-nutr-071816-064634

Pellegrini, M., Cioffi, I., Evangelista, A., Ponzo, V., Goitre, I., Ciccone, G., Ghigo, E., & Bo, S. (2020). Effects of time-restricted feeding on body weight and metabolism. A systematic review and meta-analysis. *Reviews in Endocrine and Metabolic Disorders*, 21, 17–33. https://doi.org/10.1007/s11154-019-09524-w

Pureza, I. R. O. M., Macena, M. L., da Silva, A. E. Jr., Praxedes, D. R. S., Vasconcelos, L. G. L., & Bueno, N. B. (2021). Effect of early time-restricted feeding on the metabolic profile of adults with excess weight: A systematic review with meta-analysis. *Clinical Nutrition*, 40, 1788–1799. https://doi.org/10.1016/j.clnu.2020.10.031

Schübel, R., Nattenmüller, J., Sookthai, D., Nonnenmacher, T., Graf, M. E., Riedl, L., Christopher, C. L., von Stackelberg, O., Johnson, T., Nabers, D., Kirsten, R., Kratz, M., Kauczor, H-U., Ulrich, C. M., Kaaks, R., & Kühn, T. (2018). Effects of intermittent and continuous calorie restriction on body weight and metabolism over 50 wk: A randomized controlled trial. *American Journal of Clinical Nutrition*, 108, 933–945. https://doi.org/10.1093/ajcn/nqy196

Sun, J. C., Tan, Z. T., He, C. J. Hu, H. L., Zhai, C. L., & Qian, G. (2023). Time-restricted eating with calorie restriction on weight loss and cardiometabolic risk: A systematic review and meta-analysis. *European Journal of Clinical Nutrition*, 77, 1014–1025. https://doi.org/10.1038/s41430-023-01311-w

Varady, K. A., Cienfuegos, S., Ezpeleta, M., & Gabel, K. (2022). Clinical application of intermittent fasting for weight loss: Progress and future directions. *Nature Reviews Endocrinology*, 18, 309–321. https://doi.org/10.1038/s41574-022-00638-x

Yanai, H., Park, B., Koh, H., Jang, H. J., Vaughan, K. L., Tanaka-Yano, M., Aon, M., Blanton, M., Messaoudi, I., Diaz-Ruiz, A., Mattison, J. A., & Beerman, I. (2024). Short-term periodic restricted feeding elicits metabolome-microbiome signatures with sex dimorphic persistence in primate intervention. *Nature Communications*, 15(1), 1088. https://doi.org/10.1038/s41467-024-45359-z

## SLEEP

Acuña-Castroviejo, D., Escames, G., Venegas, C., Díaz-Casado, M. E., Lima-Cabello, E., López, L. C., Rosales-Corral, S., Tan, D. X., & Reiter, R. J. (2018). Melatonin enhances NADPH synthesis in the pentose phosphate pathway in human leukocytes and erythrocytes. *Free Radical Research*, 52(7), 756–767. https://doi.org/10.1080/10715762.2018.1455823

Bekedam, A., Aartsma-Rus, A., van Putten, M., & van der Beek, E. M. (2021). Circadian regulation of redox rhythms in the hippocampus and consequences for learning and memory. *Free Radical Biology and Medicine*, 176, 47–55. https://doi.org/10.1016/j.freeradbiomed.2021.05.010

Chen, S. H., Chin, W. C., Huang, Y. S., Chuech, L. S., Lin, C. M., Lee, C. P., Lin, H. L., Tang, I., & Yeh, T. C. (2022). The effect of electromagnetic field on sleep of patients with nocturia. *Medicine*, 101(32), e29129. http://doi.org/10.1097/MD.0000000000029129

Ding, G., Gong, Y., Eckel-Mahan, K. L., & Sun, Z. (2018). Central circadian clock regulates energy metabolism. *Advances in Experimental Medicine and Biology*, 1090, 79–103. http://doi.org/10.1007/978-981-13-1286-1_5

Donga, E., van Dijk, M., van Dijk, J. G., Biermasz, N. R., Lammers, G. J., van Kralingen, K. W., Corssmit, E. P., & Romijn, J. A. (2010). A single night of partial sleep deprivation induces insulin resistance in multiple metabolic pathways in healthy subjects. *Journal of Clinical Endocrinology and Metabolism*, 95(6), 2963–2968.

Fogel, S. M., Ray, L. B., Binnie, L., & Owen, A. M. (2019). The importance of slow-wave sleep for daytime cognitive performance. *Trends in Cognitive Sciences*, 23(5), 370–383. https://doi.org/10.1016/j.tics.2019.02.004

Frantzias, J., & Doff, M. H. (2019). Mouth taping as an adjunct therapy in reducing snoring and sleep-disordered breathing. *Journal of Dental Sleep Medicine*, 6(2), 55–60.

Hatori, M., Gronfier, C., Van Reen, E., Johnson, M. P., & Klerman, E. B. (2020). Napping: A public health issue. *Sleep Medicine Reviews*, 51, 101283.

Johnson, K. G., Johnson, D. C., & Johnson, K. G. (2020). Mouth taping for sleep-disordered breathing: A review. *Journal of Clinical Sleep Medicine*, 16(7), 1163–1172.

Lee, Y. C., Lu, C. T., Cheng, W. N., & Li, H. Y. (2022). The impact of mouth-taping in mouth-breathers with mild obstructive sleep apnea: A preliminary study. *Healthcare (Basel, Switzerland)*, 10(9), 1755. https://doi.org/10.3390/healthcare10091755

Liu, S., Liu, Q., Tabuchi, M., & Wu, M. N. (2016). Sleep drive is encoded by neural plastic changes in a dedicated circuit. *Neuron*, 91(1), 25–32. https://doi.org/10.1016/j.neuron.2016.05.028

Ma, H., Deng, C., Guo, W., Guo, R., Liu, S., Zhang, Z., & Yu, M. (2018). Extremely low-frequency electromagnetic fields affect nitric oxide signaling pathway in endothelial cells: A proteomic approach. *Frontiers in Physiology*, 9, 106. http://doi.org/10.3389/fphys.2018.00106

Matsumoto, T., Kakinuma, Y., Okazaki, Y., Chikako, T., Hiroshima, M., Taniguchi, H., & Ota, T. (2021). Effect of daytime napping on glycemic control, insulin sensitivity, and β-cell function in patients with type 2 diabetes: A randomized crossover trial. *BMJ Open Diabetes Research & Care*, 9(1), e001874.

Peek, C. B., Levine, D. C., Cedernaes, J., Taguchi, A., Kobayashi, Y., Tsai, S. J., Bonar, N. A., McNulty, M. R., Ramsey, K. M., Bass, J., & Schernhammer, E. S. (2019). Circadian control of antioxidant and redox regulation in peripheral tissues. *Free Radical Biology and Medicine*, 119, 17–29. https://doi.org/10.1016/j.freeradbiomed.2018.01.036

Rihm, J. S., Menegaux, A., & Lutkenhoff, E. S. (2021). Role of slow-wave sleep in memory processing and memory-related psychiatric disorders. *Current*

*Opinion in Psychiatry*, 34(3), 242–249. https://doi.org/10.1097/YCO
.0000000000000683

Scullin, M. K., Bliwise, D. L., Perez, E., & Bliwise, N. G. (2021). Slow-wave sleep and the risk of incident Alzheimer's disease and cognitive decline in older adults. *Sleep*, 44(3), zsaa211. https://doi.org/10.1093/sleep/zsaa211

Sollott, S. J., Cheng, L., Pauly, R. R., Jenkins, G. M., Lancaster, J. R. Jr., Frazier, O. H., Ziegelstein, R. C., & Lakatta, E. G. (1995). Increased nitric oxide production during exposure to pulsed electromagnetic fields. *Biochemical and Biophysical Research Communications*, 213(3), 715–718. http://doi.org/10.1006/bbrc.1995.2210

Sutherland, K., Lee, R. W., Chan, A. S., Ng, M. T., & Cistulli, P. A. (2015). Mouth-taping during sleep: A pilot study on a new approach to reduce mouth breathing. *Sleep and Breathing*, 19(2), 611–616.

Takahashi, J. S. (2017). Transcriptional architecture of the mammalian circadian clock. *Nature Reviews Genetics*, 18(3), 164–179. http://doi.org/10.1038/nrg.2016.150

Takahashi, M., Arito, H., & Takeuchi, T. (2015). Napping during daytime disturbs human circadian rhythms of 24-hour fast-induced lipolysis and adipose gene expression. *Sleep Medicine*, 16(11), 1334–1340.

Tarullo, A. R., & Balsam, P. D. (2020). Slow wave sleep in children: Development, individual differences, and implications for brain and cognitive development. *Neuroscience & Biobehavioral Reviews*, 108, 811–824. https://doi.org/10.1016/j.neubiorev.2019.12.017

Voigt, R. M., Forsyth, C. B., & Keshavarzian, A. (2013). Circadian disruption: Potential implications in inflammatory and metabolic diseases associated with alcohol. *Alcohol Research*, 35(1), 87–96.

Westerberg, C. E., Mander, B. A., Florczak, S. M., Weintraub, S., Mesulam, M. M., Zee, P. C., & Paller, K. A. (2019). Concurrent impairments in sleep and memory in amnestic mild cognitive impairment. *Journal of the International Neuropsychological Society*, 25(2), 103–114.

Wong, J. Y. H., Liao, C. P., Lin, C. H., & Huang, C. J. (2020). Circadian regulation of NADPH oxidase activity and production of reactive oxygen species: Insights from in vivo imaging of single cells in the zebrafish. *Free Radical Biology and Medicine*, 150, 104–113. https://doi.org/10.1016/j.freeradbiomed.2020.01.009

Yamamoto, M., Tsuzuki, K., & Ogawa, Y. (2009). The effects of a mid-day nap on the glycemic response to carbohydrate-rich meals in healthy men. *Diabetes Care*, 32(11), 1916–1918.

Yoo, S. H., Yamazaki, S., Lowrey, P. L., Shimomura, K., Ko, C. H., Buhr, E. D., Siepka, S. M., Hong, H. K., Oh, W. J., Yoo, O. J., Menaker, M., & Takahashi, J. S.

(2004). PERIOD2:LUCIFERASE real-time reporting of circadian dynamics reveals persistent circadian oscillations in mouse peripheral tissues. *Proceedings of the National Academy of Sciences of the United States of America*, 101, 5339–5346.

Zielinski, M. R., McKenna, J. T., & McCarley, R. W. (2016). Functions and mechanisms of sleep. *AIMS Neuroscience*, 3(1), 67–104. http://doi.org/10.3934/Neuroscience.2016.1.67

## EXERCISE

American Heart Association. (2021). *Walking for a healthy heart.* Retrieved from https://kramesstore.com/walking-for-a-healthy-heart-aha.html

Ashrafi, H., Rafiee, G., Alizadeh, A., & Zolaktaf, V. (2021). The effects of aerobic training on cardiorespiratory fitness and quality of life in elderly people: A systematic review and meta-analysis. *Aging Clinical and Experimental Research*, 33(3), 461–469. http://doi.org/10.1007/s40520-020-01664-1

Barakat, C., & Barakat, H. (2019). Efficacy of high-intensity interval training versus moderate-intensity continuous training on cardiorespiratory fitness and body composition in sedentary adults: A systematic review and meta-analysis. *Obesity Research and Clinical Practice*, 13(6), 542–557. http://doi.org/10.1016/j.orcp.2019.09.002

Carapeto, P. V., & Aguayo-Mazzucato, C. (2021). Effects of exercise on cellular and tissue aging. *Aging*, 13(10), 14522–14543. http://doi.org/10.18632/aging.203051

Coquart, J. B., Tourny-Chollet, C., Lemaire, C., Dubart, A. E., Groslambert, A., & Tourny, C. H. (2019). Effects of a 6-week indoor cycling program on health markers in sedentary overweight adults. *Journal of Sports Medicine and Physical Fitness*, 59(2), 202–208. http://doi.org/10.23736/S0022-4707.18.08530-1

Garatachea, N., Pareja-Galeano, H., Sanchis-Gomar, F., Santos-Lozano, A., Fiuza-Luces, C., Morán, M., Emanuele, E., Joyner, M. J., & Lucia, A. (2015). Exercise attenuates the major hallmarks of aging. *Rejuvenation Research*, 18, 57–89. http://doi.org/10.1089/rej.2014.1623

Ito, S. (2019). High-intensity interval training for health benefits and care of cardiac diseases: The key to an efficient exercise protocol. *World Journal of Cardiology*, 11(7), 171–188. http://doi.org/10.4330/wjc.v11.i7.171

Kafkas, M. E., Aksu, I., & Zararsiz, G. (2021). The effect of different intensity training on plasma neopterin levels in athletes. *Journal of Clinical Laboratory Analysis*, 35(1), e23536. http://doi.org/10.1002/jcla.23536

Konttinen, N., & Kyröläinen, H. (2019). Neopterin as a potential biomarker for monitoring overreaching in athletes. *Frontiers in Physiology*, 10, 1116. http://doi.org/10.3389/fphys.2019.01116

Leng, S., Wu, Y., & Huang, W. (2020). Effects of exercise on bone mineral density in postmenopausal women with osteoporosis: A systematic review and meta-analysis. *Journal of Clinical Densitometry*, 23(3), 343–353. http://doi.org/10.1016/j.jocd.2018.10.002

Lippi, G., Sanchis-Gomar, F., Salvagno, G. L., Aloe, R., Schena, F., & Guidi, G. C. (2020). Neopterin and biopterin as diagnostic biomarkers of endurance exercise-induced stress. *Clinical Biochemistry*, 77, 54–57. http://doi.org/10.1016/j.clinbiochem.2020.01.002

Lippi, G., Schena, F., Salvagno, G. L., Aloe, R., Banfi, G., & Guidi, G. C. (2017). Neopterin and biopterin as biomarkers of overtraining. *Journal of Clinical Laboratory Analysis*, 31(6), e22121. http://doi.org/10.1002/jcla.22121

Moreira, L. D., Oliveira, M. L., Lirani-Galvão, A. P., Marin-Mio, R. V., Santos, R. N., & Lazaretti-Castro, M. (2021). Effects of resistance training on bone mineral density in women with osteoporosis or osteopenia: A systematic review with meta-analysis. *Journal of Clinical Densitometry*, 24(1), 20–29. http://doi.org/10.1016/j.jocd.2020.01.002

Woods, J. A., Wilund, K. R., Martin, S. A., & Kistler, B. M. (2012). Exercise, inflammation and aging. *Aging and Disease*, 3, 130–140.

Zhao, R., Zhao, M., Xu, Z., Liu, Y., Chen, Z., Wang, Y., & Li, Y. (2021). The effect of exercise interventions on bone mineral density in postmenopausal women with osteoporosis: A systematic review and meta-analysis. *Frontiers in Endocrinology*, 12, 728267. http://doi.org/10.3389/fendo.2021.728267

## HIIT Program

Weston, K. S., Wisloff, U., & Coombes, J. S. (2014). High-intensity interval training in patients with lifestyle-induced cardiometabolic disease: A systematic review and meta-analysis. *British Journal of Sports Medicine*, 48(16), 1227–1234. http://doi.org/10.1136/bjsports-2013-092576

## Bodyweight Program

Bhatt, T., & Ghali, F. (2021). The effect of circuit resistance training on muscular strength, endurance and body composition in adults: A systematic review and meta-analysis of randomized controlled trials. *Journal of Sports Medicine and Physical Fitness*, 61(1), 145–157. http://doi.org/10.23736/S0022-4707.20.11091-1

Colado, J. C., Garcia-Masso, X., Sanchez-Medina, L., & Triplett, N. T. (2012). Effects of a long-term resistance training program with different elastic resistance bands on anthropometry and muscular strength in sedentary older women. *Journal of Strength and Conditioning Research*, 26(4), 1130–1138. http://doi.org/10.1519/JSC.0b013e31822e5967

Colado, J. C., Garcia-Masso, X., Triplett, N. T., Calatayud, J., & Flandez, J. (2012). Concurrent validation of the OMNI-resistance exercise scale of perceived exertion with Thera-band resistance bands. *Journal of Strength and Conditioning Research*, 26(10), 2658–2664. http://doi.org/10.1519/JSC .0b013e3182443162

Cunha, P. M., Tomeleri, C. M., Nascimento, M. A., Schoenfeld, B. J., Sardinha, L. B., & Cyrino, E. S. (2019). Effect of machine-based strength training on performance in elderly women. *Experimental Gerontology*, 124, 110634. http:// doi.org/10.1016/j.exger.2019.110634

Damas, F., Phillips, S. M., Lixandrão, M. E., Vechin, F. C., Libardi, C. A., Roschel, H., & Ugrinowitsch, C. (2016). Early resistance training-induced increases in muscle cross-sectional area are concomitant with edema-induced muscle swelling. *European Journal of Applied Physiology*, 116(1), 49–56. http://doi .org/10.1007/s00421-015-3243-4

Fonseca, R. M., Roschel, H., Tricoli, V., de Souza, E. O., Wilson, J. M., Laurentino, G. C., Aihara, A. Y., de Souza Leão, A. R., & Ugrinowitsch, C. (2014). Changes in exercises are more effective than in loading schemes to improve muscle strength. *Journal of Strength and Conditioning Research*, 28(11), 3085–3092. https://doi.org/10.1519/JSC.0000000000000539

Kraemer, W. J., Ratamess, N. A., and French, D. N. (2002). Resistance training for health and performance. *Current Sports Medicine Reports*, 1(3), 165–171. https://doi.org/10.1249/00149619-200206000-00007

Neves, E. B., Colato, A. S., Ferreira, V. F., Bertani, R. F., Perez, I. A., & Ronque, E. R. (2020). Effects of circuit resistance training on body composition, functional and physiological outcomes in sedentary women: A randomized controlled trial. *European Journal of Sport Science*, 20(7), 911–919. http://doi.org /10.1080/17461391.2019.1698738

Ramirez-Campillo, R., Martinez-Salazar, C., Valdés-Badilla, P., & Izquierdo, M. (2017). Effectiveness of elastic resistance bands in rehabilitation: A systematic review and meta-analysis. *Physical Therapy in Sport*, 24, 10–22. http://doi .org/10.1016/j.ptsp.2016.07.003

Reis, V. M., Garrido, N. D., Silva, L. C., Marins, J. C., & Fernandes, H. M. (2021). Effects of bodyweight circuit training on body composition, cardiovascular fitness, and muscular strength and endurance: A systematic review and meta-analysis. *Sports Medicine*, 51(4), 743–756. http://doi.org/10.1007/s40279-020-01425-4

Rønnestad, B. R., & Mujika, I. (2014). Optimizing strength training for running and cycling endurance performance: A review. *Scandinavian Journal of Medicine & Science in Sports*, 24(4), 603–612. http://doi.org/10.1111/sms.12104

Shin, K. O., Kim, S. H., & Lee, K. R. (2018). Circuit weight training improves body composition and metabolic syndrome risk factors in obese women. *Journal of Sports Science and Medicine*, 17(4), 532–540.

Westcott, W. L., Winett, R. A., Anderson, E. S., Wojcik, J. R., Loud, R. L., Cleggett, E., & Glover, S. (2009). Effects of regular and slow speed resistance training on muscle strength. *Journal of Sports Medicine and Physical Fitness*, 49(3), 284–291.

## Visualization

Cho, H., Kim, E., & Kwon, S. (2021). Effects of imagery training on muscular strength in older adults: A systematic review and meta-analysis. *Journal of Sports Science and Medicine*, 20(3), 469–479.

Naish, M. D., & Chow, J. Y. (2021). The effects of imagery interventions on performance outcomes in strength and conditioning: A systematic review. *Journal of Strength and Conditioning Research*, 35(9), 2613–2623. http://doi.org/10.1519/JSC.0000000000004119

Whiteman-Sandland, J., Hawkins, R., Claydon-Mueller, L., & Smith, J. A. (2020). Using guided imagery to enhance perceptions of physical exertion during high-intensity interval exercise. *Medicine and Science in Sports and Exercise*, 52(2), 478–486. http://doi.org/10.1249/MSS.0000000000002144

## SUPPLEMENTS

### 1-MNA

Chudzik, M., Burzyńska, M., & Kapusta, J. (2022). Use of 1-MNA to improve exercise tolerance and fatigue in patients after COVID-19. *Nutrients*, 14(15), 3004.

European Food Safety Authority. (2017). *Safety of 1-methylnicotinamide chloride (1-MNA) as a novel food pursuant to Regulation (EC) No 258/97*. Retrieved May 6, 2024, from https://www.efsa.europa.eu/en/efsajournal/pub/5001

Sidor, K., Jeznach, A., Hoser, G., & Skirecki, T. (2023). 1-Methylnicotinamide (1-MNA) inhibits the activation of the NLRP3 inflammasome in human macrophages. *International Immunopharmacology*, 121, 110445. http://doi.org/10.1016/j.intimp.2023.110445

Song, Z., Zhong, X., Li, M., Gao, P., Ning, Z., Sun, Z., & Song, X. (2021).
1-MNA ameliorates high fat diet-induced heart injury by upregulating NRF2
expression and inhibiting NF-κb in vivo and in vitro. *Frontiers in Cardiovascular Medicine*, 8, 721814. https://doi.org/10.3389/fcvm.2021.721814

Ström, K., Morales-Alamo, D., Ottosson, F., Edlund, A., Hjort, L., Jörgensen,
S. W., Almgren, P., Zhou, Y., Martin-Rincon, M., Ekman, C., Pérez-López,
A., Ekström, O., Perez-Suarez, I., Mattiasson, M., de Pablos-Velasco, P.,
Oskolkov, N., Ahlqvist, E., Wierup, N., Eliasson, L., Vaag, A., . . . Hansson,
O. (2018). N1-methylnicotinamide is a signalling molecule produced in skeletal muscle coordinating energy metabolism. *Scientific Reports*, 8, 3016. https://doi.org/10.1038/s41598-018-21099-1

### Acetyl L-Carnitine

Álvares, T. S., Conte, C. A. Jr., Paschoalin, V. M. F., Silva, J. T., Meirelles, C. D. M.,
Bhambhani, Y. N., & Gomes, P. S. C. (2012). Acute l-arginine supplementation
increases muscle blood volume but not strength performance. *Applied Physiology, Nutrition, and Metabolism*, 37(1), 115–126. https://doi.org/10.1139/h11-144

Barrera, G., Gentile, F., Pizzimenti, S., Canuto, R. A., Daga, M., Arcaro, A.,
Cetrangolo, G. P., Lepore, A., Ferretti, C., Dianzani, C., & Muzio, G. (2016).
Mitochondrial dysfunction in cancer and neurodegenerative diseases: Spotlight on fatty acid oxidation and lipoperoxidation products. *Antioxidants (Basel, Switzerland)*, (1), 7. https://doi.org/10.3390/antiox5010007

Bergamini, E., Cavallini, G., Donati, A., & Gori, Z. (2004). The role of autophagy
in aging: Its essential part in the anti-aging mechanism of caloric restriction.
*Annals of the New York Academy of Sciences*, 1019(1), 406–411. https://doi.org/10.1196/annals.1396.020

Brandsch, C., & Eder, K. (2003). Effect of L-carnitine on weight loss and body
composition of rats fed a hypocaloric diet. *Annals of Nutrition & Metabolism*,
47(6), 241–245. http://doi.org/10.1159/000073980

Carta, A., Calvani, M., Bravi, D., & Bhuachalla, S. N. (2006). Acetyl-L-carnitine
and Alzheimer's disease: Pharmacological considerations beyond the cholinergic sphere. *Annals of the New York Academy of Sciences*, 1064(1), 228–246.
https://doi.org/10.1111/j.1749-6632.1993.tb23077.x

Cassano, P., Flück, M., Giovanna Sciancalepore, A., Pesce, V., Calvani, M.,
Hoppeler, H., Cantatore, P., & Gadaleta, M. N. (2010). Muscle unloading
potentiates the effects of acetyl-L-carnitine on the slow oxidative muscle phenotype. *BioFactors (Oxford, England)*, 36(1), 70–77. https://doi.org/10.1002/biof.74

Ferrari, R., Merli, E., Cicchitelli, G., Mele, D., Fucili, A., & Ceconi, C. (1994). Therapeutic effects of L-carnitine and propionyl-L-carnitine on cardiovascular diseases: A review. *Annals of the New York Academy of Sciences*, 719, 467–477. https://doi.org/10.1196/annals.1320.007

Hoppel, C. (2003). The role of carnitine in normal and altered fatty acid metabolism. *American Journal of Kidney Diseases*, 41(4), S4–S12. http://doi.org/10.1053/ajkd.2003.50103

Kraemer, W. J., Volek, J. S., French, D. N., Rubin, M. R., Sharman, M. J., Gómez, A. L., Ratamess, N. A., Newton, R. U., Jemiolo, B., Craig, B. W., & Häkkinen, K. (2003). The effects of L-carnitine L-tartrate supplementation on hormonal responses to resistance exercise and recovery. *Journal of Strength & Conditioning Research*, 17(3), 455–462. https://doi.org/10.1519/1533-4287(2003)017<0455:teolls>2.0.co;2

Malaguarnera, M., Bella, R., Vacante, M., Giordano, M., Malaguarnera, G., Gargante, M. P., Motta, M., Mistretta, A., Rampello, L., & Pennisi, G. (2011). Acetyl-L-carnitine reduces depression and improves quality of life in patients with minimal hepatic encephalopathy. *Scandinavian Journal of Gastroenterology*, 46(6), 750–759. https://doi.org/10.3109/00365521.2011.565067

Malaguarnera, M., Cammalleri, L., Gargante, M. P., Vacante, M., Colonna, V., & Motta, N. (2012). L-carnitine treatment reduces severity of physical and mental fatigue and increases cognitive functions in centenarians: A randomized and controlled clinical trial. *American Journal of Clinical Nutrition*, 96(5), 825–834. http://doi.org/10.3945/ajcn.111.029526

Orer, G. E., & Guzel, N. A. (2014). The effects of acute L-carnitine supplementation on endurance performance of athletes. *The Journal of Strength & Conditioning Research*, 28(2), 514–519. https://doi.org/10.1519/JSC.0b013e3182a76790

Osio, M., Muscia, F., Zampini, L., Nascimbene, C., Mailland, E., Cargnel, A., & Mariani, C. (2006). Acetyl-l-carnitine in the treatment of painful antiretroviral toxic neuropathy in human immunodeficiency virus patients: an open label study. *Journal of the Peripheral Nervous System: JPNS*, 11(1), 72–76. https://doi.org/10.1111/j.1085-9489.2006.00066.x

Ozmen, E., Ozsoy, S. Y., Donmez, N., Ozsoy, B., & Yumuşak, N. (2014). The protective effect of L-carnitine against hippocampal damage due to experimental formaldehyde intoxication in rats. *Biotechnic & Histochemistry: Official Publication of the Biological Stain Commission*, 89(5), 336–341. https://doi.org/10.3109/10520295.2013.855818

Passeri, M., Cucinotta, D., Bonati, P. A., Iannuccelli, M., Parnetti, L., & Senin, U. (1990). Acetyl-L-carnitine in the treatment of mildly demented elderly patients. *International Journal of Clinical Pharmacology Research*, 10(1–2), 75–79.

Pennisi, M., Lanza, G., Cantone, M., D'Amico, E., Fisicaro, F., Puglisi, V., Vinciguerra, L., Bella, R., Vicari, E., & Malaguarnera, G. (2020). Acetyl-L-carnitine in dementia and other cognitive disorders: A critical update. *Nutrients*, 12(5), 1389. https://doi.org/10.3390/nu12051389

Petrosillo, G., Di Venosa, N., Pistolese, M., Casanova, G., Tiravanti, E., Colantuono, G., Federici, A., Paradies, G., & Ruggiero, F. M. (2006). Protective effect of melatonin against mitochondrial dysfunction associated with cardiac ischemia- reperfusion: role of cardiolipin. *FASEB Journal: Official Publication of the Federation of American Societies for Experimental Biology*, 20(2), 269–276. https://doi.org/10.1096/fj.05-4692com

Pettegrew, J. W., Klunk, W. E., Panchalingam, K., Kanfer, J. N., & McClure, R. J. (1995). Clinical and neurochemical effects of acetyl-L-carnitine in Alzheimer's disease. *Neurobiology of Aging*, 16(1), 1–4. http://doi.org/10.1016/0197-4580(94)00120-e

Poon, H. F., Frasier, M., Shreve, N., Calabrese, V., Wolozin, B., & Butterfield, D. A. (2005). Mitochondrial associated metabolic proteins are selectively oxidized in A30P alpha-synuclein transgenic mice--a model of familial Parkinson's disease. *Neurobiology of Disease*, 18(3), 492–498. https://doi.org/10.1016/j.nbd.2004.12.009

Rosca, M. G., Vazquez, E. J., Kerner, J., Parland, W., Chandler, M. P., Stanley, W., Sabbah, H. N., & Hoppel, C. L. (2008). Cardiac mitochondria in heart failure: decrease in respirasomes and oxidative phosphorylation. *Cardiovascular Research*, 80(1), 30–39. https://doi.org/10.1093/cvr/cvn184

Sima, A. A., Calvani, M., Mehra, M., Amato, A., & Acetyl-L-Carnitine Study Group (2005). Acetyl-L-carnitine improves pain, nerve regeneration, and vibratory perception in patients with chronic diabetic neuropathy: An analysis of two randomized placebo-controlled trials. *Diabetes Care*, 28(1), 89–94. https://doi.org/10.2337/diacare.28.1.89

de Sotomayor, M. A., Mingorance, C., Rodriguez-Rodriguez, R., Marhuenda, E., & Herrera, M. D. (2007). L-carnitine and its propionate: improvement of endothelial function in SHR through superoxide dismutase-dependent mechanisms. *Free Radical Research*, 41(8), 884–891. https://doi.org/10.1080/10715760701416467

Spagnoli, A., Lucca, U., Menasce, G., Bandera, L., Cizza, G., Forloni, G., Tettamanti, M., Frattura, L., Tiraboschi, P., & Comelli, M. (1991). Long-term acetyl-L-carnitine treatment in Alzheimer's disease. *Neurology*, 41(11), 1726–1732. http://doi.org/10.1212/wnl.41.11.1726

Thal, L. J., Carta, A., Clarke, W. R., Ferris, S. H., Friedland, R. P., Petersen, R. C., Pettegrew, J. W., Pfeiffer, E., Raskind, M. A., Sano, M., Tuszynski, M. H., & Woolson, R. F. (1996). A 1-year multicenter placebo-controlled study of acetyl-L-carnitine in patients with Alzheimer's disease. *Neurology*, 47(3), 705–711. http://doi.org/10.1212/wnl.47.3.705

Traina, G. (2016). The neurobiology of acetyl-L-carnitine. *Frontiers in Bioscience*, 8, 1–17. http://doi.org/10.2741/s460

Villani, R. G., Gannon, J., Self, M., & Rich, P. A. (2000). L-carnitine supplementation combined with aerobic training does not promote weight loss in moderately obese women. *International Journal of Sports Nutrition and Exercise Metabolism*, 10(2), 199–207. http://doi.org/10.1123/ijsnem.10.2.199

Volek, J. S., Kraemer, W. J., Rubin, M. R., Gómez, A. L., Ratamess, N. A., & Gaynor, P. (2002). L-carnitine L-tartrate supplementation favorably affects markers of recovery from exercise stress. *American Journal of Physiology— Endocrinology and Metabolism*, 282(2), E474–E482. https://doi.org/10.1152 /ajpendo.00277.2001

Zammit, V. A., & Ramsay, R. R. (2002). Carnitine and its role in fatty acid metabolism. *Progress in Lipid Research*, 41(5), 361–384. http://doi.org/10.1016/s0163 -7827(02)00008-0

Zammit, V. A., Ramsay, R. R., Bonomini, M., & Arduini, A. (2006). Carnitine, mitochondrial function and therapy. *Advanced Drug Delivery Reviews*, 58(15), 1631–1650. https://doi.org/10.1016/j.addr.2009.04.024

## AKG

Bloomer, R. J., Smith, W. A., Fisher-Wellman, K. H., Oxenreider, C., & Kreider, R. B. (2007). Glycine propionyl-L-carnitine modulates lipid peroxidation and nitric oxide in human subjects. *International Journal for Vitamin and Nutrition Research*, 77(3), 131–141.

Du, J., Cullen, J. J., Buettner, G. R., & Buettner, G. R. (2012). Ascorbic acid: Chemistry, biology and the treatment of cancer. *Biochimica et Biophysica Acta*, 1826(2), 443–457.

Farsaei, S., Sadeghi-Moghaddam, B., Farahani, N., & Naderi, G. H. (2019). Alpha-ketoglutarate: Physiological functions and applications. *Biomolecules*, 9(10), 647.

Fraisl, P., & Mazzone, M. (2012). Regulation of angiogenesis by hypoxia: The role of oxygen sensing. *Journal of Developmental Biology*, 140(5), 467–474.

Gołębiowski, M., Michalski, M., & Kozłowski, R. (2020). The effect of α-ketoglutarate on the wound healing process in rats. *Journal of Veterinary Research*, 64(3), 349–356.

Huang, J., Wang, Y., Jiang, H., Frank, S. J., Lu, J., & Rosenfeld, R. G. (2017). Identification of a novel growth hormone-releasing hormone α-ketoglutarate (GHRH-AKG) responsible for improved growth hormone release in vitro and in vivo. *Molecular and Cellular Endocrinology*, 452, 64–71.

Iovine, B., Iannella, M. L., Nocella, M., Pricolo, M. R., Bevilacqua, M. A., & Capobianco, L. (2019). Mitochondrial metabolism and activity in chondrocytes of patients with osteoarthritis. *Cells*, 8(11), 1426.

Jeong, J. H., Kim, J. H., Lee, K. T., & Kim, Y. (2016). Alpha-ketoglutarate activates NRF2/ARE pathway antioxidant defense via metabolic alteration of cysteine in the 2-ketoglutarate dehydrogenase complex. *Biochimica et Biophysica Acta*, 1860(11), 2414–2424.

Jolly, C. A., Jiang, Y. H., Chapkin, R. S., & McMurray, D. N. (1993). Alpha-ketoglutarate enhances neutrophil killing activity and modulates oxidative metabolism. *Journal of Leukocyte Biology*, 54(6), 525–530.

Kaikkonen, J., Nyyssönen, K., Porkkala-Sarataho, E., Poulsen, H. E., Metsä-Ketelä, T., & Hayn, M. (2000). Effect of alpha-tocopherol and beta-carotene supplementation on cognitive functions in elderly persons. *American Journal of Clinical Nutrition*, 71(2), 829–834.

Kapahi, P., Kaeberlein, M., & Hansen, M. (2017). Dietary restriction and lifespan: Lessons from invertebrate models. *Ageing Research Reviews*, 39, 3–14.

Kim, J. W., Tchernyshyov, I., Semenza, G. L., & Dang, C. V. (2006). HIF-1-mediated expression of pyruvate dehydrogenase kinase: A metabolic switch required for cellular adaptation to hypoxia. *Cell Metabolism*, 3(3), 177–185.

Koh, J. H., Kim, J. M., Chang, U. J., Suh, H. J., & Lim, H. K. (2003). Beneficial effects of alpha-ketoglutarate on systemic inflammation and multiple organ dysfunction syndrome induced by endotoxemia in rats. *Journal of Surgical Research*, 111(2), 218–226.

Lee, S. J., Kim, H. G., Lee, S. J., Chang, K. C., & Kim, J. K. (2019). The anti-aging properties of a synthetic functional compound, AG-CS10, extracted from the leaves of Panax ginseng. *Molecules*, 24(15), 2706.

Li, M., Li, X., Zhang, H., Lu, Y., Li, X., & Xia, H. (2016). Alpha-ketoglutarate inhibits glutamine degradation and enhances protein synthesis in hepatocytes of blunt snout bream (*Megalobrama amblycephala*) fed a low-protein diet. *Scientific Reports*, 6, 31012.

Liu, S., He, L., & Yao, K. (2018). The antioxidative function of alpha-ketoglutarate and its applications. *BioMed Research International*, 2018, 3408467. https://doi.org/10.1155/2018/3408467

Mero, A. A., Ojala, T., Hulmi, J. J., Puurtinen, R., Karila, T. A., Seppälä, T., & Kallio, P. (2010). Effects of alfa-hydroxy-isocaproic acid on body composition, DOMS and performance in athletes. *Journal of the International Society of Sports Nutrition*, 7(1), 1–7.

Ra, S. G., Miyazaki, T., Ishikura, K., Nagayama, H., Suzuki, T., Maeda, S., Ito, M., Matsuzaki, Y., & Ohmori, H. (2013). Additional effects of taurine on the benefits of BCAA intake for the delayed-onset muscle soreness and muscle damage induced by high-intensity eccentric exercise. *Advances in Experimental Medicine and Biology*, 776, 179–187. https://doi.org/10.1007/978-1-4614-6093-0_18

Selak, M. A., Armour, S. M., MacKenzie, E. D., Boulahbel, H., Watson, D. G., Mansfield, K. D., Pan, Y., Simon, M. C., Thompson, C. B., & Gottlieb, E. (2005). Succinate links TCA cycle dysfunction to oncogenesis by inhibiting HIF-α prolyl hydroxylase. *Cancer Cell*, 7(1), 77–85. https://doi.org/10.1016/j.ccr.2004.11.022

Semenza, G. L. (2003). Targeting HIF-1 for cancer therapy. *Nature Reviews Cancer*, 3(10), 721–732.

Sharma, R., Kumar, P., & Chakraborty, S. (2016). Alpha-ketoglutarate suppresses the NF-κB-mediated oxidative stress pathway for attenuating colonic inflammation in dextran sulfate sodium-induced experimental colitis. *Journal of Microbiology and Biotechnology*, 26(9), 1545–1552.

Shimomura, Y., Murakami, T., Nakai, N., Nagasaki, M., & Harris, R. A. (2004). Exercise promotes BCAA catabolism: Effects of BCAA supplementation on skeletal muscle during exercise. *Journal of Nutrition*, 134(6 Suppl), 1583S–1587S.

Sugino, T., Shirai, T., Kajimoto, Y., & Kajimoto, O. (2008). L-ornithine supplementation attenuates physical fatigue in healthy volunteers by modulating lipid and amino acid metabolism. *Nutrition Research*, 28(11), 738–743.

Sun, Y., Xu, Y., Xu, J., Wu, Z., Wu, T., & Zhang, Y. (2020). Dietary α-ketoglutarate supplementation enhances immune status in a mouse model of intrauterine growth restriction. *British Journal of Nutrition*, 123(4), 439–447.

Xu, J., Liu, Y., Li, Y., Wang, X., Yang, H., Zhang, Q., & Shi, W. (2018). The beneficial effects of α-ketoglutarate on skeletal muscle in aged mice: Role of uncoupling protein 2 and AMP-activated protein kinase signaling. *International Journal of Molecular Sciences*, 19(6), 1810.

Yamamoto, N., Soga, T., & Hattori, K. (2019). Mental and physical fatigue-related biochemical alterations. *Nutrition*, 60, 112–117.

Yang, M., Kim, J., Kim, J. H., Kim, H. E., Lee, J., & Moon, E. Y. (2013). Alpha-ketoglutarate attenuates the lipopolysaccharide-induced production of inflammatory mediators in BV2 microglial cells. *Journal of Functional Foods*, 5(4), 1747–1755.

Yu, L., Li, Y., Li, Y., Zhao, J., & Li, L. (2019). Effects of α-ketoglutarate on energy metabolism in hippocampal neurons under hypoxia. *Brain Research*, 1704, 23–29.

## Bicarbonate

Boron, W. F., & Boulpaep, E. L. (2009). *Medical physiology: A cellular and molecular approach*. Elsevier Health Sciences.

Carr, A. J., Slater, G. J., & Gore, C. J. (2011). Effects of sodium bicarbonate on prolonged intermittent exercise. *Medicine and Science in Sports and Exercise*, 43(5), 821–829.

Dawson-Hughes, B., Harris, S. S., & Ceglia, L. (2008). Alkaline diets favor lean tissue mass in older adults. *American Journal of Clinical Nutrition*, 87(3), 662–665.

Dawson-Hughes, B., Harris, S. S., Palermo, N. J., Castaneda-Sceppa, C., Rasmussen, H. M., & Dallal, G. E. (2009). Treatment with potassium bicarbonate lowers calcium excretion and bone resorption in older men and women. *Journal of Clinical Endocrinology and Metabolism*, 94(1), 96–102.

de Brito-Ashurst, I., Varagunam, M., Raftery, M. J., & Yaqoob, M. M. (2009). Bicarbonate supplementation slows progression of CKD and improves nutritional status. *Journal of the American Society of Nephrology*, 20(9), 2075–2084.

DiBaise, J. K., & Crowell, M. D. (2013). Role of bicarbonate therapy in digestive diseases. *Mayo Clinic Proceedings*, 88(4), 414–426.

Foster, M. W., & McMahon, T. J. (2013). S-nitrosylation in health and disease: Trends and mechanisms. *Nature Reviews Molecular Cell Biology*, 14(2), 142–156.

Frassetto, L. A., Todd, K. M., Morris, R. C., & Sebastian, A. (2000). Worldwide incidence of hip fracture in elderly women: Relation to consumption of animal and vegetable foods. *Journal of Gerontology*, 55(10), M585–M592.

Ganceviciene, R., Liakou, A. I., Theodoridis, A., Makrantonaki, E., & Zouboulis, C. C. (2012). Skin anti-aging strategies. *Dermato-Endocrinology*, 4(3), 308–319.

Ghosh, S., Chisti, Y., & Banerjee, U. C. (2012). Production of shikimic acid. *Biotechnology Advances*, 30(6), 1425–1431.

Gill, R. K., Saksena, S., Alrefai, W. A., Sarwar, Z., Goldstein, J. L., Carroll, R. E., Ramaswamy, K., & Dudeja, P. K. (2005). Expression and membrane localization of MCT isoforms along the length of the human intestine. *American Journal of Physiology – Gastrointestinal and Liver Physiology*, 289(4), G711–G722.

Kemi, V. E., Kärkkäinen, M. U., Rita, H. J., Laaksonen, M. M., Outila, T. A., & Lamberg-Allardt, C. J. (2010). Low calcium:phosphorus ratio in habitual diets affects serum parathyroid hormone concentration and calcium metabolism in healthy women with adequate calcium intake. *British Journal of Nutrition*, 103(4), 561–568.

Lelli, M., Putignano, A., Marchetti, M., Foltran, I., Mangani, F., Procaccini, M., Roveri, N., & Orsini, G. (2010). Remineralization and repair of enamel surface by biomimetic Zn-carbonate hydroxyapatite containing toothpaste: A comparative in vivo study. *Frontiers in Physiology*, 5, 333. https://doi.org/10.3389/fphys.2014.00333

Macdonald, H. M., Black, A. J., Aucott, L., Duthie, G., Duthie, S., Sandison, R., Hardcastle, A. C., Lanham-New, S. A., Fraser, W. D., & Reid, D. M. (2008). Effect of potassium citrate supplementation or increased fruit and vegetable intake on bone metabolism in healthy postmenopausal women: A randomized controlled trial. *American Journal of Clinical Nutrition*, 88(2), 465–474.

McNaughton, L. R., Ford, S., Newbold, C., & Richardson, M. (1996). The effects of sodium bicarbonate ingestion on exercise performance. *Journal of Sports Sciences*, 14(3), 165–171.

Mizock, B. A. (2000). The role of bicarbonate therapy in lactic acidosis. *Chest*, 117(1), 260–267.

Peart, D. J., & Siegler, J. C. (2011). Bicarbonate supplementation and its effects on anaerobic exercise performance: A meta-analysis. *Journal of Strength and Conditioning Research*, 25(4), 1109–1117.

Sale, C., Saunders, B., Hudson, S., Wise, J. A., Harris, R. C., & Sunderland, C. D. (2011). Effect of β-alanine plus sodium bicarbonate on high-intensity cycling capacity. *Medicine and Science in Sports and Exercise*, 43(10), 1972–1978.

Sebastian, A., Frassetto, L. A., Sellmeyer, D. E., & Morris, R. C. Jr. (2002). The acid-base effects of bone resorption and formation in humans. *Journal of Bone and Mineral Research*, 17(4), 741–747.

Siegler, J. C., Marshall, P. W., & Raftry, S. (2013). Effect of sodium bicarbonate supplementation on repeated sprints during intermittent exercise performed in hypoxia. *Journal of Strength and Conditioning Research*, 27(2), 450–458.

Wang, Y., Xie, Z., Wang, Y., Wang, Z., Zhang, J., Tian, J., Chen, X., & Zhu, Z. (2013). Amelioration of oxidative stress and apoptosis: A neuroprotective role for hydrogen sulfide in traumatic brain injury. *Brain Research*, 1517, 129–137.

Wynn, E., Krieg, M. A., Aeschlimann, J. M., & Burckhardt, P. (2004). Alkaline mineral supplementation decreases bone resorption in postmenopausal women with osteopenia. *Journal of Bone and Mineral Research*, 19(4), 558–566.

## Bovine Colostrum

Bagwe-Parab, S., Yadav, P., Kaur, G., Tuli, H. S., & Buttar, H. S. (2020). Therapeutic applications of human and bovine colostrum in the treatment of gastrointestinal diseases and distinctive cancer types: The current evidence. *Frontiers in Pharmacology*, 11, 01100. https://www.frontiersin.org/articles/10.3389/fphar.2020.01100

Dziewiecka, H., Buttar, H. S., Kasperska, A., Ostapiuk-Karolczuk, J., Domagalska, M., Cichoń, J., & Skarpańska-Stejnborn, A. (2022). A systematic review of the influence of bovine colostrum supplementation on leaky gut syndrome in athletes: Diagnostic biomarkers and future directions. *Nutrients*, 14(12), 2512. https://doi.org/10.3390/nu14122512

Guberti, M., Botti, S., Capuzzo, M. T., Nardozi, S., Fusco, A., Cera, A., Dugo, L., Piredda, M., & De Marinis, M. G. (2021). Bovine colostrum applications in sick and healthy people: A systematic review. *Nutrients*, 13(7), 2194. https://doi.org/10.3390/nu13072194

## Butyrate

Arpaia, N., Campbell, C., Fan, X., Dikiy, S., van der Veeken, J., deRoos, P., Liu, H., Cross, J. R., Pfeffer, K., Coffer, P. J., & Rudensky, A. Y. (2013). Metabolites produced by commensal bacteria promote peripheral regulatory T-cell generation. *Nature*, 504(7480), 451–455. http://doi.org/10.1038/nature12726

Bhattarai, Y., Muniz Pedrogo, D. A., & Kashyap, P. C. (2017). Irritable bowel syndrome: A gut microbiota-related disorder?. *American Journal of Physiology – Gastrointestinal and Liver Physiology*, 312(1), G52–G62. http://doi.org/10.1152/ajpgi.00338.2016

Bindels, L. B., Delzenne, N. M., Cani, P. D., & Walter, J. (2015). Towards a more comprehensive concept for prebiotics. *Nature Reviews Gastroenterology & Hepatology*, 12(5), 303–310. http://doi.org/10.1038/nrgastro.2015.47

Canani, R. B., Costanzo, M. D., Leone, L., Pedata, M., Meli, R., & Calignano, A. (2011). Potential beneficial effects of butyrate in intestinal and extraintestinal diseases. *World Journal of Gastroenterology*, 17(12), 1519–1528. http://doi.org/10.3748/wjg.v17.i12.1519

Canfora, E. E., Jocken, J. W., & Blaak, E. E. (2015). Short-chain fatty acids in control of body weight and insulin sensitivity. *Nature Reviews Endocrinology*, 11(10), 577–591. http://doi.org/10.1038/nrendo.2015.128

Canfora, E. E., van der Beek, C. M., Jocken, J. W. E., Goossens, G. H., Holst, J. J., Olde Damink, S. W. M., Lenaerts, K., Dejong, C. H. C., & Blaak, E. E. (2017). Colonic infusions of short-chain fatty acid mixtures promote energy metabolism in overweight/obese men: A randomized crossover trial. *Scientific Reports*, 7(1), 2360. https://doi.org/10.1038/s41598-017-02546-x

Chandra-Hioe, M. V., Wong, C. H., & Arcot, J. (2017). The potential use of beta-glucans from cereal milling by-products as functional food ingredients. *Journal of the Science of Food and Agriculture*, 97(3), 684–692. http://doi.org/10.1002/jsfa.7824

Cummings, N. E., Williams, E. M., Kasza, I., Konon, E. N., Schaid, M. D., Schmidt, B. A., Poudel, C., Sherman, D. S., Yu, D., Arriola Apelo, S. I., Cottrell, S. E., Geiger, G., Barnes, M. E., Wisinski, J. A., Fenske, R. J., Matkowskyj, K. A., Kimple, M. E., Alexander, C. M., Merrins, M. J., & Lamming, D. W. (2018). Restoration of metabolic health by decreased consumption of branched-chain amino acids. *Journal of Physiology*, 596(4), 623–645. http://doi.org/10.1113/JP275075

Dahiya, D. K., Renuka, P., Shandilya, U. K., Dhewa, T. (2021). Butyrate: A potent tool for microbiome manipulation and therapeutic applications. *Critical*

*Reviews in Food Science and Nutrition*, 61(16), 2677–2695. http://doi.org/10.10 80/10408398.2020.1723613

Davie, J. R. (2003). Inhibition of histone deacetylase activity by butyrate. *Journal of Nutrition*, 133(7 Suppl), 2485S–2493S. http://doi.org/10.1093/jn/133 .7.2485S

Fu, L., Zhang, G., Qian, S., Zhang, Q., & Tan, M. (2022). Associations between dietary fiber intake and cardiovascular risk factors: An umbrella review of meta-analyses of randomized controlled trials. *Frontiers in Nutrition*, 9. https://doi.org/10.3389/fnut.2022.972399

Gérard, P. (2016). Gut microbiota and obesity. *Cellular and Molecular Life Sciences*, 73(1), 147–162. http://doi.org/10.1007/s00018-015-2061-5

Govindarajan, B., & Gipson, I. K. (2011). Short-chain fatty acids, butyrate and propionate, regulate gene expression and function of the human intestinal epithelium. *International Journal of Toxicology*, 30(6), 603–620. http://doi.org /10.1177/1091581811420179

Guo, T.-T., Zhang, Z., Sun, Y., Zhu, R.-Y., Wang, F.-X., Ma, L.-J., Jiang, L., & Liu, H.-D. (2023). Neuroprotective effects of sodium butyrate by restoring gut microbiota and inhibiting TLR4 signaling in mice with MPTP-induced Parkinson's disease. *Nutrients* 15(4), 930. https://doi.org/10.3390/nu 15040930

Haenen, D., Zhang, J., Souza da Silva, C., Bosch, G., van der Meer, I. M., van Arkel, J., van den Borne, J. J., Pérez Gutiérrez, O., Smidt, H., Kemp, B., Müller, M., & Hooiveld, G. J. (2013). A diet high in resistant starch modulates microbiota composition, SCFA concentrations, and gene expression in pig intestine. *Journal of Nutrition*, 143(3), 274–283. https://doi.org/10.3945 /jn.112.169672

Henningsson, A., Marsh, J. A., Lonnerdal, B., Hernell, O., & Domellof, M. (2014). Effects of dietary fiber intake on inflammation in critically ill children. *Journal of Parenteral and Enteral Nutrition*, 38(7), 811–818. http://doi.org /10.1177/0148607114523482

Kim, C. H., Park, J., & Kim, M. (2014). Gut microbiota-derived short-chain fatty acids, T cells, and inflammation. *Immune Network*, 14(6), 277–288. http://doi .org/10.4110/in.2014.14.6.277

Kim, H., Kim, Y., & Kwon, O. (2017). Beneficial effects of butyrate on increasing insulin sensitivity in relation to energy metabolism via intracellular mechanism. *Asian-Australasian Journal of Animal Sciences*, 30(12), 1710–1719. http:// doi.org/10.5713/ajas.17.0434

Kim, S. W., Park, K. Y., Kim, B., Kim, E., & Hyun, C. K. (2017). Butyrate enhances muscle mass and reduces body fat in broiler chickens. *Asian-Australasian Journal of Animal Sciences*, 30(12), 1782–1787. http://doi.org/10.5713/ajas.17.0295

Kimura, I., Ozawa, K., Inoue, D., Imamura, T., Kimura, K., Maeda, T., Terasawa, K., Kashihara, D., Hirano, K., Tani, T., Takahashi, T., Miyauchi, S., Shioi, G., Inoue, H., & Tsujimoto, G. (2013). The gut microbiota suppresses insulin-mediated fat accumulation via the short-chain fatty acid receptor GPR43. *Nature Communications*, 4, 1829. http://doi.org/10.1038/ncomms2852

Li, H., He, J., & Jia, W. (2016). The influence of gut microbiota on drug metabolism and toxicity. *Expert Opinion on Drug Metabolism & Toxicology*, 12(1), 31–40. http://doi/org/10.1517/17425255.2016.1120119

Li, H., Zhang, L., Li, J., Wu, Q., Qian, L., He, J., Ni, Y., Kovatcheva-Datchary, P., Yuan, R., Liu, S., Shen, L., Zhang, M., Sheng, B., Li, P., Kang, K., Wu, L., Fang, Q., Long, X., Wang, X., Li, Y., . . . Jia, W. (2024). Resistant starch intake facilitates weight loss in humans by reshaping the gut microbiota. *Nature Metabolism*, 6(3), 578–597. https://doi.org/10.1038/s42255-024-00988-y

Li, Q., Cao, L., Tian, Y., Zhang, P., Ding, C., Lu, W., Jia, C., Shao, C., Liu, W., Wang, D., Ye, H., & Hao, H. (2018). Butyrate suppresses the proliferation of colorectal cancer cells via targeting pyruvate kinase M2 and metabolic reprogramming. *Molecular & Cellular Proteomics: MCP*, 17(8), 1531–1545. https://doi.org/10.1074/mcp.RA118.000752

Lin, H. V., Frassetto, A., Kowalik, E. J., Jr., Nawrocki, A. R., Lu, M. M., Kosinski, J. R., Hubert, J. A., Szeto, D., Yao, X., Forrest, G., & Marsh, D. J. (2012). Butyrate and propionate protect against diet-induced obesity and regulate gut hormones via free fatty acid receptor 3-independent mechanisms. *PloS One*, 7(4), e35240. https://doi.org/10.1371/journal.pone.0035240

Lührs, H., Gerke, T., Müller, J. G., Melcher, R., Schauber, J., Boxberge, F., Scheppach, W., & Menzel, T. (2002). Butyrate inhibits NF-kappaB activation in lamina propria macrophages of patients with ulcerative colitis. *Scandinavian Journal of Gastroenterology*, 37(4), 458–466. https://doi.org/10.1080/003655202317316105

McRae, M. P. (2014). Beta-glucan from barley and its lipid-lowering capacity: A review of clinical trials. *Annals of Nutrition and Metabolism*, 64(2), 96–107. http://doi.org/10.1159/000356328

Murray, R. L., Zhang, W., Liu, J., Cooper, J., Mitchell, A., Buman, M., Song, J., & Stahl, C. H. (2021). Tributyrin, a butyrate pro-drug, primes satellite cells for differentiation by altering the epigenetic landscape. *Cells*, 10(12), 3475. https://doi.org/10.3390/cells10123475

Park, B., Kim, J., Riffey, O., Dowker-Key, P., Bruckbauer, A., McLoughlin, J., Bettaieb, A., & Donohoe, D. (2022). Pyruvate kinase m1 regulates butyrate metabolism in cancerous colonocytes. *Scientific Reports*, 12, 8771. https://doi.org/10.1038/s41598-022-12827-9

Ramirez-Farias, C., Slezak, K., Fuller, Z., Duncan, A., Holtrop, G., & Louis, P. (2009). Effect of inulin on the human gut microbiota: Stimulation of *Bifidobacterium adolescentis* and *Faecalibacterium prausnitzii*. *British Journal of Nutrition*, 101(4), 541–550. http://doi.org/10.1017/S0007114508019880

Recharla, N., Geesala, R., & Shi, X-J. (2023). Gut microbial metabolite butyrate and its therapeutic role in inflammatory bowel disease: A literature review. *Nutrients*, 15(10), 2275. https://doi.org/10.3390/nu15102275

Sivaprakasam, S., Bhutia, Y. D., Yang, S., & Ganapathy, V. (2017). Short-chain fatty acid transporters: Role in colonic homeostasis. *Comprehensive Physiology*, 8(1), 299–314. http://doi.org/10.1002/cphy.c170011

Suzuki, T., Yoshida, S., & Hara, H. (2008). Physiological concentrations of short-chain fatty acids immediately suppress colonic epithelial permeability. *British Journal of Nutrition*, 100(2), 297–305. http://doi.org/10.1017/S0007114508888736

van der Beek, C. M., Bloemen, J. G., van den Broek, M. A., Lenaerts, K., Venema, K., Buurman, W. A., & Dejong, C. H. (2015). Hepatic uptake of rectally administered butyrate prevents an increase in systemic butyrate concentrations in humans. *Journal of Nutrition*, 145(9), 2019–2024. https://doi.org/10.3945/jn.115.211193

Vernia, P., Marcheggiano, A., Caprilli, R., Frieri, G., Corrao, G., Valpiani, D., Di Paolo, M. C., Paoluzi, P., & Torsoli, A. (1995). Short-chain fatty acid topical treatment in distal ulcerative colitis. *Alimentary Pharmacology & Therapeutics*, 9(3), 309–313. https://doi.org/10.1111/j.1365-2036.1995.tb00386.x

Wilms, E., Jonkers, D. M. A. E., Savelkoul, H. F. J., Elizalde, M., Tischmann, L., de Vos, P., Masclee, A. A. M., & Troost, F. J. (2019). The impact of pectin supplementation on intestinal barrier function in healthy young adults and healthy elderly. *Nutrients*, 11(7), 1554. https://doi.org/10.3390/nu11071554

Yang, J., Summanen, P. H., Henning, S. M., Hsu, M., Lam, H., Huang, J., Tseng, C. H., Dowd, S. E., Finegold, S. M., Heber, D., & Li, Z. (2015). Xylooligosaccharide supplementation alters gut bacteria in both healthy and prediabetic adults: A pilot study. *Frontiers in Physiology*, 6, 216. https://doi.org/10.3389/fphys.2015.00216

Zeng, H., Umar, S., Rust, B., Lazarova, D., & Bordonaro, M. (2019). Secondary bile acids and short chain fatty acids in the colon: A focus on colonic microbiome, cell proliferation, inflammation, and cancer. *International Journal of Molecular Sciences*, 20(21), E5542. http://doi.org/10.3390/ijms20215542


## Collagen Peptides

Chen, Q., Chen, O., Martins, I., Hou, H., Zhao, X, Blumberg, J., & Li, B. (2017). Collagen peptides ameliorate intestinal epithelial barrier dysfunction in immunostimulatory caco-2 cell monolayers via enhancing tight junctions. *Food & Function*, 8(3): 1144–51. https://doi.org/10.1039/C6FO01347C

Elango, J., Zamora-Ledezma, C., Ge, B., Hou, C., Pan, Z., Bao, B., Pérez Albacete Martínez, C., Granero Marín, J. M., de Val, J. E. M. S., Bao, C., & Wu, W. (2022). Paradoxical duel role of collagen in rheumatoid arthritis: Cause of inflammation and treatment. *Bioengineering (Basel, Switzerland)*, 9(7), 321. https://doi.org/10.3390/bioengineering9070321

König, D., Oesser, S., Scharla, S., Zdzieblik, D., & Gollhofer, A. (2018). Specific collagen peptides improve bone mineral density and bone markers in post-menopausal women—a randomized controlled study. *Nutrients*, 10(1), 97. https://doi.org/10.3390/nu10010097

Martínez-Puig, D., Costa-Larrión, E., Rubio-Rodríguez, N., & Gálvez-Martín, P. (2023). Collagen supplementation for joint health: The link between composition and scientific knowledge. *Nutrients*, 15(6), 1332. https://doi.org/10.3390/nu15061332

McAlindon, T. E., Nuite, M., Krishnan, N., Ruthazer, R., Price, L. L., Burstein, D., Griffith, J., & Flechsenhar, K. (2011). Change in knee osteoarthritis cartilage detected by delayed gadolinium enhanced magnetic resonance imaging following treatment with collagen hydrolysate: A pilot randomized controlled trial. *Osteoarthritis and Cartilage*, 19(4), 399–405. https://doi.org/10.1016/j.joca.2011.01.001

Nishikimi, A., Koyama, Y. I., Ishihara, S., Kobayashi, S., Tometsuka, C., Kusubata, M., Kuwaba, K., Hayashida, O., Hattori, S., & Katagiri, K. (2018). Collagen-derived peptides modulate CD4[+] T-cell differentiation and suppress allergic responses in mice. *Immunity, Inflammation and Disease*, 6(2), 245–255. https://doi.org/10.1002/iid3.213

Niu, X. Deng,S., Li, S., Xi, Y., Li, C., Wang, L., He, D., Wang, Z., & Chen, G. (2016). Therapeutic effect of ergotope peptides on collagen-induced arthritis by downregulation of inflammatory and Th1/Th17 responses and induction of regulatory T cells. *Molecular Medicine*, 22(1), 608–20. https://doi.org/10.2119/molmed.2015.00182

Proksch, E., Schunck, M., Zague, V., Segger, D., Degwert, J., & Oesser, S. (2014). Oral intake of specific bioactive collagen peptides reduces skin wrinkles and increases dermal matrix synthesis. *Skin Pharmacology and Physiology*, 27(3), 113–119. http://doi.org/10.1159/000355523

Proksch, E., Segger, D., Degwert, J., Schunck, M., Zague, V., & Oesser, S. (2014). Oral supplementation of specific collagen peptides has beneficial effects on human skin physiology: A double-blind, placebo-controlled study. *Skin Pharmacology and Physiology*, 27(1), 47–55. http://doi.org/10.1159/000351376

Schunck, M., Zague, V., Oesser, S., & Proksch, E. (2015). Dietary supplementation with specific collagen peptides has a body mass index-dependent beneficial effect on cellulite morphology. *Journal of Medicinal Food*, 18(12), 1340–1348. http://doi.org/10.1089/jmf.2015.0022

Tanaka, M., Koyama, Y., & Nomura, Y. (2015). Effects of collagen peptide ingestion on the skin. *Journal of Aging Research & Clinical Practice*, 7(5), 438–443. http://doi.org/10.1007/s12079-015-0297-5

Tanaka, M., Koyama, Y. I., & Nomura, Y. (2009). Effects of collagen peptide ingestion on UV-B-induced skin damage. *Bioscience, Biotechnology, and Biochemistry*, 73(4), 930–932. https://doi.org/10.1271/bbb.80649

Zdzieblik, D., Oesser, S., Gollhofer, A., & König, D. (2017). Improvement of activity-related knee joint discomfort following supplementation of specific collagen peptides. *Applied Physiology, Nutrition, and Metabolism*, 42(6), 588–595. http://doi.org/10.1139/apnm-2016-0390

Zhang, Z., Wang, J., Ding, Y., Dai, X., & Li, Y. (2011). Oral administration of marine collagen peptides from Chum Salmon skin enhances cutaneous wound healing and angiogenesis in rats. *Journal of the Science of Food and Agriculture*, 91(12), 2173–2179. https://doi.org/10.1002/jsfa.4435

Zhang, Z., Zhu, H., Zheng, Y., Zhang, L., Wang, X., Luo, Z., Tang, J., Lin, L., Du, Z., & Dong, C. (2020). The effects and mechanism of collagen peptide and elastin peptide on skin aging induced by D-galactose combined with ultraviolet radiation. *Journal of Photochemistry and Photobiology. B, Biology*, 210, 111964. https://doi.org/10.1016/j.jphotobiol.2020.111964

Zheng, F., Fornoni, A., Elliot, S. J., Guan, Y., Breyer, M. D., Striker, L. J., & Striker, G. E. (2002). Upregulation of type I collagen by TGF-beta in mesangial cells is blocked by PPARgamma activation. *American Journal of Physiology. Renal Physiology*, 282(4), F639–F648. https://doi.org/10.1152/ajprenal.00189.2001

## Creatine

Andres, R. H., Ducray, A. D., Schlattner, U., Wallimann, T., & Widmer, H. R. (2008). Functions and effects of creatine in the central nervous system. *Brain Research Bulletin*, 76(4), 329–343.

Béard, E., Braissant, O., Torrent, C., Henry, H., & Eichler, M. (2011). Creatine supplementation and age influence muscle metabolism and exercise tolerance in tg mice overexpressing the creatine transporter. *Journal of Applied Physiology*, 110(3), 746–754.

Böning, D., Maassen, N., Pfüller, B., & Fink, G. A. (1998). Influence of creatine supplementation on metabolite levels in aging humans. *Acta Physiologica Scandinavica*, 164(2), 147–155.

Brosnan, J. T., & Brosnan, M. E. (2007). Creatine: Endogenous metabolite, dietary, and therapeutic supplement. *Annual Review of Nutrition*, 27, 241–261.

Brosnan, J. T., & Brosnan, M. E. (2016). Creatine: Endogenous metabolite, dietary, and therapeutic supplement. *Annual Review of Nutrition*, 36, 401–417.

Buford, T., Kreider, R., Stout, J., Greenwood, M., Campbell, B., Spano, M., Ziegenfuss, T., Lopez, H., Landis, J., & Antonio, J. (2007). International Society of Sports nutrition position stand: creatine supplementation and exercise. *Journal of the International Society of Sports Nutrition*, 4(1), 6. https://doi.org/10.1186/1550-2783-4-6

Cooper, R., Naclerio, F., Allgrove, J., & Jimenez, A. (2012). Creatine supplementation with specific view to exercise/sports performance: An update. *Journal of the International Society of Sports Nutrition*, 9(1), 33.

Dechent, P., Pouwels, P. J., Wilken, B., Hanefeld, F., & Frahm, J. (1999). Increase of total creatine in human brain after oral supplementation of creatine-monohydrate. *American Journal of Physiology – Regulatory, Integrative and Comparative Physiology*, 277(3), R698–R704.

Deldicque, L., & Francaux, M. (2008). Potential harmful effects of dietary supplements in sports medicine. *Current Opinion in Clinical Nutrition and Metabolic Care*, 11(5), 610–614.

Gualano, B., Rawson, E. S., Candow, D. G., & Chilibeck, P. D. (2016). Creatine supplementation in the aging population: Effects on skeletal muscle, bone and brain. *Amino Acids*, 48(8), 1793–1805.

Jäger, R., Purpura, M., Shao, A., Inoue, T., & Kreider, R. B. (2011). Analysis of the efficacy, safety, and regulatory status of novel forms of creatine. *Amino Acids*, 40(5), 1369–1383.

Kreider, R. B., Kalman, D. S., Antonio, J., Ziegenfuss, T. N., Wildman, R., Collins, R., Candow, D. G., Kleiner, S. M., Almada, A. L., & Lopez, H. L. (2017). International Society of Sports Nutrition position stand: Safety and efficacy of creatine supplementation in exercise, sport, and medicine. *Journal of the International Society of Sports Nutrition*, 14, 18. https://doi.org/10.1186/s12970-017-0173-z

Lawler, J. M., Barnes, W. S., Wu, G., Song, W., & Demaree, S. (2002). Direct antioxidant properties of creatine. *Biochemical and Biophysical Research Communications*, 290(1), 47–52.

McMorris, T., Mielcarz, G., Harris, R. C., Swain, J. P., & Howard, A. (2007). Creatine supplementation and cognitive performance in elderly individuals. *Aging, Neuropsychology, and Cognition*, 14(5), 517–528.

Mujika, I., & Padilla, S. (2001). Creatine supplementation as an ergogenic aid for sports performance in highly trained athletes: A critical review. *International Journal of Sports Medicine*, 22(5), 378–386.

Peeters, B. M., Lantz, C. D., Mayhew, J. L., & Ware, J. S. (1999). Effect of oral creatine monohydrate and creatine phosphate supplementation on maximal strength indices, body composition, and blood pressure. *Journal of Strength and Conditioning Research*, 13(1), 3–9.

Persky, A. M., & Brazeau, G. A. (2001). Clinical pharmacology of the dietary supplement creatine monohydrate. *Pharmacological Reviews*, 53(2), 161–176.

Rawson, E. S., & Volek, J. S. (2003). Effects of creatine supplementation and resistance training on muscle strength and weightlifting performance. *Journal of Strength and Conditioning Research*, 17(4), 822–831.

Roitman, S., Green, T., Osher, Y., Karni, N., & Levine, J. (2007). Creatine monohydrate in resistant depression: Preliminary results. *Clinical Neuropharmacology*, 30(5), 307–316.

Santos, R. V., Bassit, R. A., Caperuto, E. C., & Costa Rosa, L. F. (2004). The effect of creatine supplementation upon inflammatory and muscle soreness markers after a 30km race. *Life Sciences*, 75(16), 1917–1924.

Stuerenburg, H. J., & Kunze, K. (2003). Concentrations of creatine, creatinine, and carnitine in various brain regions of patients with Alzheimer's disease. *Journal of Neural Transmission*, 110(6), 723–730.

van der Aa, M. P., & Kompier, M. A. (2019). Creatine as a therapeutic strategy for maintaining cellular energy homeostasis in neurodegenerative diseases. *Frontiers in Neuroscience*, 13, 768.

## Epicatechin

Davison, G., Callister, R., Williamson, G., Cooper, K. A., & Gleeson, M. (2012). The effect of acute pre-workout supplementation on power and strength performance. *Journal of the International Society of Sports Nutrition*, 9(1), 1–10.

Decroix, L., Tonoli, C., Soares, D. D., Tagougui, S., Heyman, E., Meeusen, R., & Piacentini, M. F. (2016). Acute cocoa flavanol improves cerebral oxygenation without enhancing executive function at rest or after exercise. *Applied Physiology, Nutrition, and Metabolism*, 41(12), 1225–1232.

Flammer, A. J., Sudano, I., Wolfrum, M., Thomas, R., Enseleit, F., Périat, D., Kaiser, P., Hirt, A., Hermann, M., Serafini, M., Lévêques, A., Lüscher, T. F., Ruschitzka, F., Noll, G., & Corti, R. (2012). Cardiovascular effects of flavanol-rich chocolate in patients with heart failure. *European Heart Journal*, 33(17), 2172–2180. https://doi.org/10.1093/eurheartj/ehr448

Gu, Y., Lambert, J. D., Chin, K. V., & Sang, S. (2011). Cocoa flavanol derivatives exhibit antiproliferative activity against human breast cancer cells. *Journal of Agricultural and Food Chemistry*, 59(18), 9878–9883.

Hammerstone, J. F., Lazarus, S. A., Mitchell, A. E., Rucker, R., Schmitz, H. H., & Toma, R. B. (2000). Identification of procyanidins in cocoa (Theobroma cacao) and chocolate using high-performance liquid chromatography/mass spectrometry. *Journal of Agricultural and Food Chemistry*, 48(10), 5320–5325.

Hooper, L., Kay, C., Abdelhamid, A., & Kroon, P. A. (2012). Effects of chocolate, cocoa, and flavan-3-ols on cardiovascular health: A systematic review and meta-analysis of randomized trials. *American Journal of Clinical Nutrition*, 95(3), 740–751.

Katz, D. L., Doughty, K., & Ali, A. (2011). Cocoa and chocolate in human health and disease. *Antioxidants and Redox Signaling*, 15(10), 2779–2811.

Khan, N., Khymenets, O., Urpí-Sardà, M., Tulipani, S., Garcia-Aloy, M., Monagas, M., Mora-Cubillos, X., Llorach, R., & Andres-Lacueva, C. (2014). Cocoa polyphenols and inflammatory markers of cardiovascular disease. *Nutrients*, 6(2), 844–880. https://doi.org/10.3390/nu6020844

Natsume, M., Osakabe, N., Yamagishi, M., Takizawa, T., Nakamura, T., Miyatake, H., Hatano, T., & Yoshida, T. (2000). Analyses of polyphenols in cacao liquor, cocoa, and chocolate by normal-phase and reversed-phase HPLC. *Bioscience, biotechnology, and biochemistry*, 64(12), 2581–2587. https://doi.org/10.1271/bbb.64.2581

Ramirez-Sanchez, I., Maya, L., Ceballos, G., & Villarreal, F. (2008). (-)-Epicatechin induces calcium and translocation independent eNOS activation in arterial endothelial cells. *American Journal of Physiology – Cell Physiology*, 294(2), C601–C607.

Rodriguez-Mateos, A., & Heiss, C. (2014). Cocoa polyphenols and cardiovascular disease: Effects on endothelial and platelet function. *Archives of Biochemistry and Biophysics*, 559, 10–14.

Scholey, A., & Owen, L. (2013). Effects of chocolate on cognitive function and mood: A systematic review. *Nutrition Reviews*, 71(10), 665–681.

Schroeter, H., Heiss, C., Balzer, J., Kleinbongard, P., Keen, C. L., Hollenberg, N. K., Sies, H., Kwik-Uribe, C., Schmitz, H. H., & Kelm, M. (2006). (-)-Epicatechin mediates beneficial effects of flavanol-rich cocoa on vascular function in humans. *Proceedings of the National Academy of Sciences of the United States of America*, 103(4), 1024–1029. https://doi.org/10.1073/pnas.0510168103

Selmi, C., Cocchi, C. A., Lanfredini, M., Keen, C. L., & Gershwin, M. E. (2016). Chocolate at heart: The anti-inflammatory impact of cocoa flavanols. *Molecular Nutrition & Food Research*, 60(8), 1756–1759.

Shukitt-Hale, B., Miller, M. G., Chu, Y. F., Lyle, B. J., Joseph, J. A., & Greenberg, J. A. (2015). Cocoa flavanols and brain perfusion. *Journal of Cardiovascular Pharmacology*, 66(4), 338–348.

Sun, X., Liu, J., Cao, X., & Sun, X. (2018). Epicatechin gallate improves insulin resistance in high fat diet-induced obese mice. *Biomedicine & Pharmacotherapy*, 101, 691–696.

**Ketone Esters**

Clarke, K., Tchabanenko, K., Pawlosky, R., Carter, E., Todd King, M., Musa-Veloso, K., & Ho, M. (2012). Kinetics, safety and tolerability of (R)-3-hydroxybutyl (R)-3-hydroxybutyrate in healthy adult subjects. *Regulatory Toxicology and Pharmacology*, 63(3), 401–408.

Evans, M., Patchett, E., Nally, R., Kearns, R., Larney, M., Egan, B., & Gearhart, J. (2017). Effect of acute ingestion of β-hydroxybutyrate salts on the response to graded exercise in trained cyclists. *European Journal of Sport Science*, 17(4), 506–513.

Murray, A. J., Knight, N. S., Cole, M. A., Cochlin, L. E., Carter, E., Tchabanenko, K., Pichulik, T., Gulston, M. K., Atherton, H. J., Schroeder, M. A., Deacon, R. M., Kashiwaya, Y., King, M. T., Pawlosky, R., Rawlins, J. N., Tyler, D. J., Griffin, J. L., Robertson, J., Veech, R. L., & Clarke, K. (2016). Novel ketone diet enhances physical and cognitive performance. *FASEB journal: Official publication of the Federation of American Societies for Experimental Biology*, 30(12), 4021–4032. https://doi.org/10.1096/fj.201600773R

Newport, M. T., VanItallie, T. B., Kashiwaya, Y., King, M. T., & Veech, R. L. (2015). A new way to produce hyperketonemia: Use of ketone ester in a case of Alzheimer's disease. *Alzheimer's & Dementia*, 11(1), 99–103.

O'Malley, T., Myette-Cote, E., Durrer, C., & Little, J. P. (2017). Nutritional ketone salts increase fat oxidation but impair high-intensity exercise performance in healthy adult males. *Applied Physiology, Nutrition, and Metabolism*, 42(10), 1031–1035.

Oosthuyse, T., & Carstens, M. (2014). Long-term administration of ketone esters attenuates renal injury in rats subjected to oxidative stress during hyperbaric oxygen exposure. *Experimental Physiology*, 99(7), 1055–1067.

Rodger, S., Plews, D., Laursen, P. B., & Driller, M. W. (2017). Oral β-hydroxybutyrate salt fails to improve 4-minute cycling performance following submaximal exercise. *Journal of the International Society of Sports Nutrition*, 14(1), 44.

Soto-Mota, A., Vansant, H., Evans, R. D., & Clarke, K. (2019). Safety and tolerability of sustained exogenous ketosis using ketone monoester drinks for 28 days in healthy adults. *Regulatory Toxicology and Pharmacology*, 109, 104506.

Stubbs, B. J., Cox, P. J., Evans, R. D., Santer, P., Miller, J. J., Faull, O. K., Magor-Elliott, S., Hiyama, S., Stirling, M., & Clarke, K. (2017). On the Metabolism of Exogenous Ketones in Humans. *Frontiers in Physiology*, 8, 848. https://doi.org/10.3389/fphys.2017.00848

**Lactulose**

Bouhnik, Y., Vahedi, K., Achour, L., Attar, A., Salfati, J., Pochart, P., Marteau, P., Flourié, B., Bornet, F., & Rambaud, J. C. (1999). Short-chain fructo-oligosaccharide administration dose-dependently increases fecal bifidobacteria in healthy humans. *Journal of Nutrition*, 129(1), 113–116. https://doi.org/10.1093/jn/129.1.113

Cani, P. D., & Delzenne, N. M. (2007). The role of the gut microbiota in energy metabolism and metabolic disease. *Current Pharmaceutical Design*, 13(21), 2173–2182.

Cho, S. S., & Finocchiaro, E. T. (Eds.). (2018). *Handbook of prebiotics and probiotics ingredients*. CRC Press.

Cryan, J. F., & Dinan, T. G. (2012). Mind-altering microorganisms: The impact of the gut microbiota on brain and behaviour. *Nature Reviews Neuroscience*, 13(10), 701–712.

Martín-Sánchez, A. M., Cuesta, I., Collado, M. C., & Hernández-Chirlaque, C. (2021). Prebiotic lactulose as a potential modulator of the gut microbial ecology against oxidative stress. *Food & Function*, 12(12), 5375–5393. https://doi .org/10.1039/d1fo00832c

Mavrogeni, M. E., Asadpoor, M., Henricks, P. A., Keshavarzian, A., Folkerts, G., & Braber, S. (2022). Direct action of non-digestible oligosaccharides against a leaky gut. *Nutrients*, 14(21), 4699. https://doi.org/10.3390/nu14214699

MedlinePlus. (2022). *Lactulose.* Retrieved May 6, 2024, from https://medlineplus. gov/druginfo/meds/a682338.html

Merrifield, C. A., Lewis, M. C., & Berger, B. (2016). Prebiotic fiber modulation of the gut microbiota improves risk factors for obesity and the metabolic syndrome. *Gut Microbes*, 7(2), 146–153.

Nicolucci, A. C., Hume, M. P., Martínez, I., Mayengbam, S., Walter, J., & Reimer, R. A. (2017). Prebiotic reduces body fat and alters intestinal microbiota in children with overweight or obesity. *Gastroenterology*, 153(3), 711–722.

Roberfroid, M. B. (2007). Prebiotics: The concept revisited. *Journal of Nutrition*, 137(3), 830S–837S.

Shukla, P. K., Meena, A. S., Dalal, R., & Shrivastava, A. (2018). Lactulose: An indirect antioxidant. *Journal of Clinical and Diagnostic Research*, 12(4), FF01. https://doi.org/10.7860/JCDR/2018/34513.11347

Tao, Y., Drabik, K. A., Waypa, T. S., Musch, M. W., Alverdy, J. C., & Schneewind, O. (2006). Soluble factors from Lactobacillus GG activate MAPKs and induce cytoprotective heat shock proteins in intestinal epithelial cells. *American Journal of Physiology – Gastrointestinal and Liver Physiology*, 290(4), G871–G878.

## L-Carnosine

Babizhayev, M. A., & Yegorov, Y. E. (2006). Telomere attrition in human lens epithelial cells associated with oxidative stress provide a new therapeutic target for the treatment, dissolving and prevention of cataract with N-acetyl-carnosine lubricant eye drops. Kinetic and mechanistic studies involving the safeguarding DNA integrity, molecular chaperone protection and transfection of the damaged DNA with the hTERT gene. *Current Drug Metabolism*, 7(6), 677–696. http://doi.org/10.2174/138920006779010332

Baguet, A., Bourgois, J., Vanhee, L., Achten, E., & Derave, W. (2010). Important role of muscle carnosine in rowing performance. *Journal of Applied Physiology*, 109(4), 1096–1101. http://doi.org/10.1152/japplphysiol.00141.2010

Baguet, A., Reyngoudt, H., Pottier, A., Everaert, I., Callens, S., & Achten, E. (2009). Carnosine loading and washout in human skeletal muscles. *Journal of Applied Physiology*, 106(3), 837–842. http://doi.org/10.1152/japplphysiol .91357.2008

Barski, L., & Jurczak, T. (2021). Carnosine in medicine: An update of biochemical and clinical research. *European Journal of Pharmacology*, 898, 173988. http:// doi.org/10.1016/j.ejphar.2021.173988

Baye, E., & Ukropec, J. (2017). Carnosine: Can understanding its actions on energy metabolism and protein homeostasis inform its therapeutic potential?. *Chemistry Central Journal*, 11(1), 1–11. http://doi.org/10.1186/s13065-017 -0304-7

Boldyrev, A. A., Aldini, G., & Derave, W. (2013). Physiology and pathophysiology of carnosine. *Physiological Reviews*, 93(4), 1803–1845. http://doi.org/10.1152 /physrev.00039.2012

Gallant, S., Kukley, M., Staubli, U., & Rush, R. A. (2004). Localization of car-nosine-like immunoreactivity in the rat brain. *Brain Research*, 1026(1), 53–59. http://doi.org/10.1016/j.brainres.2004.08.003

Hipkiss, A. R. (2007). Could carnosine or related structures suppress Alzheimer's disease? *Journal of Alzheimer's Disease*, 11(2), 229–240. http://doi.org/10.3233 /JAD-2007-11209

Hipkiss, A. R. (2012). Carnosine and its possible roles in nutrition and health. *Advances in Food and Nutrition Research*, 67, 1–52. http://doi.org/10.1016 /B978-0-12-394598-3.00001-6

Kaur, S., & Rana, P. (2020). Carnosine: An effective anti-aging molecule. *Austin Journal of Clinical Pathology*, 7(1), 1134.

Kong, X. Y., Mathias, R., & Kim, J. (2015). The role of carnosine in the modula-tion of the immune system. *Life Sciences*, 136, 41–46. http://doi.org/10.1016 /j.lfs.2015.07.016

Li, Y., Xie, Y., Li, X., Ma, X., & Jin, Y. (2019). Effects of L-carnosine on oxidative stress in isolated mouse pancreatic islets. *Journal of Diabetes Research*, 2019, 1–9. https://doi.org/10.1016/j.mce.2018.02.016

Pekar, T., & Neniskyte, U. (2020). Recent advances in the neurobiology of carnosine and its possible role in neuroprotection. *Molecular and Cellular Neuroscience*, 109, 103573. http://doi.org/10.1016/j.mcn.2020.103573

Shao, Y., He, T., Fisher, G. J., Voorhees, J. J., & Quan, T. (2017). Molecular basis of retinol anti-aging properties in naturally aged human skin in vivo. *International Journal of Cosmetic Science*, 39(1), 56–65. http://doi.org/10.1111/ics.12350

Stohs, S. J., & Badmaev, V. (2021). A review of natural dietary carnosine research in human and animal physiology. *Journal of Dietary Supplements*, 18(5), 616–639. http://doi.org/10.1080/19390211.2021.1933607

Wu, Y., Li, X., Zhu, J., Xie, Y., & Luo, X. (2022). Carnosine in health and disease: A review. *Frontiers in Physiology*, 13, 785456. http://doi.org/10.3389/fphys.2022.785456

## L-Citrulline

Bailey, S. J., Blackwell, J. R., Lord, T., Vanhatalo, A., Winyard, P. G., & Jones, A. M. (1985). L-citrulline supplementation improves O2 uptake kinetics and high-intensity exercise performance in humans. *Journal of Applied Physiology*, 119(9), 385–395. http://doi.org/10.1152/japplphysiol.00192.2014

Cormio, L., De Siati, M., Lorusso, F., Selvaggio, O., Mirabella, L., Sanguedolce, F., & Carrieri, G. (2011). Oral L-citrulline supplementation improves erection hardness in men with mild erectile dysfunction. *Urology*, 77(1), 119–122. http://doi.org/10.1016/j.urology.2010.08.028

El-Hattab, A. W., Emrick, L. T., Chanprasert, S., Craigen, W. J., & Scaglia, F. (2012). Citrulline and arginine utility in treating nitric oxide deficiency in mitochondrial disorders. *Molecular Genetics and Metabolism*, 107(3), 247–252. http://doi.org/10.1016/j.ymgme.2012.07.019

Figueroa, A., Trivino, J. A., Sanchez-Gonzalez, M. A., & Vicil, F. (2010). Oral L-citrulline supplementation attenuates blood pressure response to cold pressor test in young men. *American Journal of Hypertension*, 23(1), 12–16. http://doi.org/10.1038/ajh.2009.193

Figueroa, A., Wong, A., Jaime, S. J., & Gonzales, J. U. (2017). Influence of L-citrulline and watermelon supplementation on vascular function and exercise performance. *Current Opinion in Clinical Nutrition & Metabolic Care*, 20(1), 92–98. http://doi.org/10.1097/MCO.0000000000000340

Morita, M., Hayashi, T., Ochiai, M., Maeda, M., Yamaguchi, T., Ina, K., & Kuzuya, M. (2014). Oral supplementation with a combination of L-citrulline and L-arginine rapidly increases plasma L-arginine concentration and enhances NO bioavailability. *Biochemical and Biophysical Research Communications*, 454(4), 53–57. http://doi.org/10.1016/j.bbrc.2014.09.020

Ochiai, M., Hayashi, T., Morita, M., Ina, K., Maeda, M., Watanabe, F., & Morishita, K. (2012). Short-term effects of L-citrulline supplementation on arterial stiffness in middle-aged men. *International Journal of Cardiology*, 155(2), 257–261. http://doi.org/10.1016/j.ijcard.2010.10.004

Pérez-Guisado, J., & Jakeman, P. M. (2010). Citrulline malate enhances athletic anaerobic performance and relieves muscle soreness. *Journal of Strength and Conditioning Research*, 24(5), 1215–1222. http://doi.org/10.1519/JSC.0b013e3181cb28e0

Schwedhelm, E., Maas, R., Freese, R., Jung, D., Lukacs, Z., Jambrecina, A., Spickler, W., Schulze, F., & Böger, R. H. (2008). Pharmacokinetic and pharmacodynamic properties of oral L-citrulline and L-arginine: Impact on nitric oxide metabolism. *British Journal of Clinical Pharmacology*, 65(1), 51–59. http://doi.org/10.1111/j.1365-2125.2007.02990.x

Wu, G., Bazer, F. W., Davis, T. A., Kim, S. W., Li, P., Marc Rhoads, J., Carey Satterfield, M., Smith, S. B., Spencer, T. E., & Yin, Y. (2009). Arginine metabolism and nutrition in growth, health and disease. *Amino Acids*, 37(1), 153–168. http://doi.org/10.1007/s00726-008-0210-y

Zhang, M., Izumi, I., Kagamimori, S., Sokejima, S., Yamagami, T., Liu, Z., & Qi, B. (2004). Role of taurine supplementation to prevent exercise-induced oxidative stress in healthy young men. *Amino Acids*, 26(2), 203–207. http://doi.org/10.1007/s00726-003-0018-2

## Lithium Orotate

Baethge, C. (2020). Low-dose lithium against dementia. *International Journal of Bipolar Disorders*, 8(1), 25. https://doiorg/10.1186/s40345-020-00188-z

Chandra, S. (2021). Low-*dose lithium supplements for mental health*. Retrieved May 6, 2024, from https://chandramd.com/low-dose-lithium-supplements

Fang, Y., Chen, B., Liu, Z., Gong, A. Y., Gunning, W. T., Ge, Y., Malhotra, D., Gohara, A. F., Dworkin, L. D., & Gong, R. (2022). Age-related GSK3β overexpression drives podocyte senescence and glomerular aging. *Journal of Clinical Investigation*, 132(4), e141848. https://doi.org/10.1172/JCI141848

Forlenza, O. V., Radanovic, M., Talib, L. L., & Gattaz, W. F. (2019). Clinical and biological effects of long-term lithium treatment in older adults with amnestic mild cognitive impairment: Randomised clinical trial. *British Journal of Psychiatry*, 215(5), 668–674. https://doi.org/10.1192/bjp.2019.76

Hamstra, S. I., Roy, B. D., Tiidus, P., MacNeil, A. J., Klentrou, P., MacPherson, R. E. K., & Fajardo, V. A. (2023). Beyond its psychiatric use: The benefits of low-dose lithium supplementation. *Current Neuropharmacology*, 21(4), 891–910. https://doi.org/10.2174/1570159X20666220302151224

Huang, S., Hu, S., Liu, S., Tang, B., Liu, Y., Tang, L., Lei, Y., Zhong, L., Yang, S., & He, S. (2022). Lithium carbonate alleviates colon inflammation through modulating gut microbiota and TReg cells in a GPR43-dependent manner. *Pharmacological Research*, 175, 105992. https://doi.org/10.1016/j.phrs.2021.105992

Pacholko, A. G., & Bekar, L. K. (2021). Lithium orotate: A superior option for lithium therapy? *Brain and Behavior*, 11(8), e2262. https://doi.org/10.1002/brb3.2262

Post, R. M. (2018). The new news about lithium: An underutilized treatment in the United States. *Neuropsychopharmacology*, 43(5), 1174–1179. https://doi.org/10.1038/npp.2017.238

Shim, S. S., Berglund, K., & Yu, S. P. (2023). Lithium: An old drug for new therapeutic strategy for Alzheimer's disease and related dementia. *Neurodegenerative Diseases*, 23(1-2), 1–12. https://doi.org/10.1159/000533797

University of Toledo. (2022). *Low-dose lithium may slow kidney aging*. Retrieved July 23, 2022, from https://www.sciencedaily.com/releases/2022/04/220412095324.htm

Viel, T., Chinta, S., Rane, A., Chamoli, M., Buck, H., & Andersen, J. (2020). Microdose lithium reduces cellular senescence in human astrocytes: A potential pharmacotherapy for COVID-19?. *Aging*, 12(11), 10035–10040. https://doi.org/10.18632/aging.103449

Voytovych, H., Kriváneková, L., & Ziemann, U. (2012). Lithium: A switch from LTD- to LTP-like plasticity in human cortex. *Neuropharmacology*, 63(2), 274–279. https://doi.org/10.1016/j.neuropharm.2012.03.023


## L-Leucine

Blomstrand, E., Eliasson, J., Karlsson, H. K., & Köhnke, R. (2006). Branched-chain amino acids activate key enzymes in protein synthesis after physical exercise. *Journal of Nutrition*, 136(1 Suppl), 269S–273S. http://doi.org/10.1093/jn/136.1.269S

Churchward-Venne, T. A., Burd, N. A., Mitchell, C. J., West, D. W., Philp, A., Marcotte, G. R., Baker, S. K., Baar, K., & Phillips, S. M. (2012). Supplementation of a suboptimal protein dose with leucine or essential amino acids: Effects on myofibrillar protein synthesis at rest and following resistance exercise in men. *Journal of Physiology*, 590(11), 2751–2765. https://doi.org/10.1113/jphysiol.2012.228833

Hirschey, M. D., Shimazu, T., Goetzman, E., Jing, E., Schwer, B., Lombard, D. B., Grueter, C. A., Harris, C., Biddinger, S., Ilkayeva, O. R., Stevens, R. D., Li, Y., Saha, A. K., Ruderman, N. B., Bain, J. R., Newgard, C. B., Farese, R. V. Jr.,

Alt, F. W., Kahn, C. R., & Verdin, E. (2010). SIRT3 regulates mitochondrial fatty-acid oxidation by reversible enzyme deacetylation. *Nature*, 464(7285), 121–125. https://doi.org/10.1038/nature08778

Holeček, M. (2018). Branched-chain amino acids in health and disease: Metabolism, alterations in blood plasma, and as supplements. *Nutrition & Metabolism*, 15(1), 33. http://doi.org/10.1186/s12986-018-0271-1

Katsanos, C. S., Kobayashi, H., Sheffield-Moore, M., Aarsland, A., & Wolfe, R. R. (2006). A high proportion of leucine is required for optimal stimulation of the rate of muscle protein synthesis by essential amino acids in the elderly. *Journal of Nutrition*, 136(5), 1262–1267. http://doi.org/10.1093/jn/136.5.1262

Matsumoto, K., Koba, T., Hamada, K., Sakurai, M., Higuchi, T., & Miyata, H. (2009). Branched-chain amino acid supplementation increases the lactate threshold during an incremental exercise test in trained individuals. *Journal of Nutritional Science and Vitaminology*, 55(1), 52–58. http://doi.org/10.3177/jnsv.55.52

Matthews, J. J., & Zachwieja, J. J. (2017). Nutrient composition of meat. In *Encyclopedia of Food and Health* (pp. 19–24). Academic Press.

Nairizi, A., She, P., Vary, T. C., & Lynch, C. J. (2009). Leucine supplementation of drinking water does not alter susceptibility to diet-induced obesity in mice. *Journal of Nutrition*, 139(1), 95–100. http://doi.org/10.3945/jn.108.095901

Ochiai, M., Matsuo, T., Suzuki, Y., Hasegawa, T., & Miyata, H. (2012). Short-term effects of L-citrulline supplementation on arterial stiffness in middle-aged men. *International Journal of Cardiology*, 155(2), 257–261. http://doi.org/10.1016/j.ijcard.2010.09.057

Park, S. J., Ahmad, F., Philp, A., Baar, K., Williams, T., Luo, H., Ke, H., Rehmann, H., Taussig, R., Brown, A. L., Kim, M. K., Beaven, M. A., Burgin, A. B., Manganiello, V., & Chung, J. H. (2012). Resveratrol ameliorates aging-related metabolic phenotypes by inhibiting cAMP phosphodiesterases. *Cell*, 148(3), 421–433. https://doi.org/10.1016/j.cell.2012.01.017

Phillips, S. M., & Van Loon, L. J. (2011). Dietary protein for athletes: From requirements to optimum adaptation. *Journal of Sports Sciences*, 29(sup1), S29–S38. http://doi.org/10.1080/02640414.2011.619204

Rieu, I., Balage, M., Sornet, C., Giraudet, C., Pujos, E., Grizard, J., Mosoni, L., & Dardevet, D. (2006). Leucine supplementation improves muscle protein synthesis in elderly men independently of hyperaminoacidaemia. *Journal of Physiology*, 575(Pt 3), 845–855. https://doi.org/10.1113/jphysiol.2006.110742

Ryu, D., Mouchiroud, L., Andreux, P. A., Katsyuba, E., Moullan, N., Nicolet-Dit-Félix, A. A., Williams, E. G., Jha, P., Lo Sasso, G., Huzard, D., Aebischer, P., Sandi, C., Rinsch, C., & Auwerx, J. (2016). Urolithin A induces mitophagy and prolongs lifespan in C. elegans and increases muscle function in rodents. *Nature Medicine*, 22(8), 879–888. https://doi.org/10.1038/nm.4132

USDA FoodData Central. (n.d.). Search results for "Cheese, cheddar". Retrieved March 31, 2023, from https://fdc.nal.usda.gov/fdc-app.html#/food-details /168468/nutrients

USDA FoodData Central. (n.d.). Search results for "Chicken, broilers or fryers, breast, meat only, raw". Retrieved March 31, 2023, from https://fdc.nal.usda .gov/fdc-app.html#/food-details/172425/nutrients

USDA FoodData Central. (n.d.). Search results for "Nuts, almonds". Retrieved March 31, 2023, from https://fdc.nal.usda.gov/fdc-app.html#/food-details /171262/nutrients

USDA FoodData Central. (n.d.). Search results for "Soybeans, mature seeds, raw". Retrieved March 31, 2023, from https://fdc.nal.usda.gov/fdc-app.html# /food-details/169513/nutrients

Verhoeven, S., Vanschoonbeek, K., Verdijk, L. B., Koopman,. R, Wodzig, W. K., Dendale, P., & van Loon, L. J. (2009). Long-term leucine supplementation does not increase muscle mass or strength in healthy elderly men. *American Journal of Clinical Nutrition*, 90(1), 705–713. http://doi.org/10.3945/ajcn .2008.27231

Zemel, M. B. (2020). Modulation of energy sensing by leucine synergy with natural sirtuin activators: Effects on health span. *Journal of Medicinal Food*, 23(11), 1129–1135. https://doi.org/10.1089/jmf.2020.0105

Zhang, L., Li, F., Guo, Q., Duan, Y., Wang, W., Zhong, Z., Yang, Y., & Yin, Y. (2020). Leucine supplementation: A novel strategy for modulating lipid metabolism and energy homeostasis. *Nutrients*, 12(5), 1299. https://doi.org/10 .3390/nu12051299

Zhou, Z., Yin, H., Guo, Y., Fang, Y., Yuan, F., Chen, S., & Guo, F. (2021). A fifty percent leucine-restricted diet reduces fat mass and improves glucose regulation. *Nutrition & Metabolism*, 18(1), 34. https://doi.org/10.1186/s12986 -021-00564-1

## L-Theanine

Dietz, C., & Dekker, M. (2017). Effect of green tea phytochemicals on mood and cognition. *Current Pharmaceutical Design*, 23(19), 2876–2905. http://doi.org/1 0.2174/1381612823666170105151141

Egashira, N., Ishigami, N., Pu, F., Mishima, K., Iwasaki, K., Orito, K., Oishi, R., & Fujiwara, M. (2008). Theanine prevents memory impairment induced by repeated cerebral ischemia in rats. *Phytotherapy Research: PTR*, 22(1), 65–68. https://doi.org/10.1002/ptr.2261

Einöther, S. J., Martens, V. E., Rycroft, J. A., & De Bruin, E. A. (2010). L-theanine and caffeine improve task switching but not intersensory attention or subjective alertness. *Appetite*, 54(2), 406–409. https://doi.org/10.1016/j.appet.2010.01.003

Higashiyama, A., Htay, H. H., Ozeki, M., & Juneja, L. R. (2011). Effects of L-theanine on attention and reaction time response. *Journal of Functional Foods*, 3(3), 171–178. http://doi.org/10.1016/j.jff.2011.03.009

Jang, H. S., Jung, J. Y., Jang, I. S., & Jang, K. H. (2016). L-theanine partially counteracts caffeine-induced sleep disturbances in rats. *Pharmacology Biochemistry and Behavior*, 145, 24–30. http://doi.org/10.1016/j.pbb.2016.03.009

Kim, H. J., Kim, Y. J., Lee, S. Y., Jeong, S. M., & Lee, J. H. (2017). The neuroprotective effects of theanine: A possible role in neurodegenerative diseases. *Journal of Clinical Neurology*, 13(4), 385–393. http://doi.org/10.3988/jcn.2017.13.4.385

Kim, T. I., Lee, Y. K., Park, S. G., Choi, I. S., Ban, J. O., Park, H. K., Nam, S. Y., Yun, Y. W., Han, S. B., Oh, K. W., & Hong, J. T. (2009). l-Theanine, an amino acid in green tea, attenuates beta-amyloid-induced cognitive dysfunction and neurotoxicity: reduction in oxidative damage and inactivation of ERK/p38 kinase and NF-kappaB pathways. *Free Radical Biology & Medicine*, 47(11), 1601–1610. https://doi.org/10.1016/j.freeradbiomed.2009.09.008

Kimura, K., Ozeki, M., Juneja, L. R., & Ohira, H. (2007). L-theanine reduces psychological and physiological stress responses. *Biological Psychology*, 74(1), 39–45. http://doi.org/10.1016/j.biopsycho.2006.06.006

Lu, K., Gray, M. A., Oliver, C., Liley, D. T., Harrison, B. J., Bartholomeusz, C. F., Phan, K. L., & Nathan, P. J. (2004). The acute effects of L-theanine in comparison with alprazolam on anticipatory anxiety in humans. *Human Psychopharmacology*, 19(7), 457–465. https://doi.org/10.1002/hup.611

Lyon, M. R., Kapoor, M. P., & Juneja, L. R. (2011). The effects of L-theanine (Suntheanine®) on objective sleep quality in boys with attention deficit hyperactivity disorder (ADHD): A randomized, double-blind, placebo-controlled clinical trial. *Alternative Medicine Review*, 16(4), 348–354.

Matsuguma, M., Miyata, Y., Kusano, Y., & Uchida, K. (2019). L-theanine elicits an immune-stimulatory response in vitro and in vivo. *Phytotherapy Research*, 33(6), 1637–1645. http://doi.org/10.1002/ptr.6374

Nagai, K., Oda, A., & Konishi, H. (2015). Theanine prevents doxorubicin-induced acute hepatotoxicity by reducing intrinsic apoptotic response. *Food and Chemical Toxicology: An International Journal Published for the British Industrial Biological Research Association*, 78, 147–152. https://doi.org/10.1016/j.fct.2015.02.009

Nakamura, H., Ukawa, Y., & Sakagami, H. (2004). Binding of glutathione to the tea polyphenol, (-)-epigallocatechin gallate, through cysteine in rat digestive tract. *Bioscience, Biotechnology, and Biochemistry*, 68(4), 957–959.

Rao, T. P., Ozeki, M., & Juneja, L. R. (2015). In search of a safe natural sleep aid. *Journal of the American College of Nutrition*, 34(5), 436–447. http://doi.org/10.1080/07315724.2014.926153

Siamwala, J. H., Dias, P. M., Majumder, S., Joshi, M. K., Sinkar, V. P., Banerjee, G., & Chatterjee, S. (2013). L-theanine promotes nitric oxide production in endothelial cells through eNOS phosphorylation. *Journal of Nutritional Biochemistry*, 24(3), 595-605. https://doi.org/10.1016/j.jnutbio.2012.02.016

Unno, K., Tanida, N., Ishii, N., Yamamoto, H., Iguchi, K., Hoshino, M., Takeda, A., Ozawa, H., Ohkubo, T., Juneja, L. R., & Yamada, H. (2013). Anti-stress effect of theanine on students during pharmacy practice: Positive correlation among salivary α-amylase activity, trait anxiety and subjective stress. *Pharmacology, Biochemistry, and Behavior*, 111, 128–135. https://doi.org/10.1016/j.pbb.2013.09.004

Wiegant, F. A., Surinova, S., Ytsma, E., Langelaar-Makkinje, M., Wikman, G., & Post, J. A. (2009). Plant adaptogens increase lifespan and stress resistance in *C. elegans*. *Biogerontology*, 10(1), 27–42. http://doi.org/10.1007/s10522-008-9151-9

Yokogoshi, H., Kobayashi, M., Mochizuki, M., & Terashima, T. (1998). Effect of theanine, r-glutamylethylamide, on brain monoamines and striatal dopamine release in conscious rats. *Neurochemical Research*, 23(5), 667–673. http://doi.org/10.1023/A:1022490806095

Yokogoshi, H., Mochizuki, M., & Saitoh, K. (1998). Theanine-induced reduction of brain serotonin concentration in rats. *Bioscience, Biotechnology, and Biochemistry*, 62(4), 816–817. http://doi.org/10.1271/bbb.62.816

## L-Tryptophan

Alkhatib, N., & Atcheson, J. M. (2020). L-tryptophan: Basic metabolic functions, behavioral research and therapeutic indications. *International Journal of Tryptophan Research*, 13, 1–16. https://doi.org/10.1177/1178646920917376

Badawy, A. A.-B. (2017). Kynurenine pathway of tryptophan metabolism: Regulatory and functional aspects. *International Journal of Tryptophan Research*, 10, 1178646917691938. https://doi.org/10.1177/1178646917691938

Bhatti, J., & Gillin, J. C. (2014). Serotonin and sleep. *Sleep Medicine Clinics*, 9(1), 13–29. https://doi.org/10.1016/j.jsmc.2013.10.002

Birdsall, T. C. (1998). 5-Hydroxytryptophan: A clinically-effective serotonin precursor. *Alternative Medicine Review*, 3(4), 271–280. https://pubmed.ncbi.nlm.nih.gov/9727088

Chen, Y., Lu, J., Huang, Y., Wang, T., Xu, Y., Xu, M., & Chen, L. (2018). L-tryptophan activates NRF2-dependent antioxidant response and protects against oxidative damage in endothelial cells. *Biochemical and Biophysical Research Communications*, 498(4), 946–952. https://doi.org/10.1016/j.bbrc.2018.03.091

Chyan, Y.-J., Poeggeler, B., Omar, R. A., Chain, D. G., Frangione, B., Ghiso, J., & Pappolla, M. A. (1999). Potent neuroprotective properties against the

Alzheimer beta-amyloid by an endogenous melatonin-related indole structure, indole-3-propionic acid. *Journal of Biological Chemistry*, 274(31), 21937–21942. https://doi.org/10.1074/jbc.274.31.21937

De Pergola, G., & Silvestris, F. (2013). Obesity as a major risk factor for cancer. *Journal of Obesity*, 2013, 291546. https://doi.org/10.1155/2013/291546

Halbreich, U., Bergeron, R., Yonkers, K., Freeman, E., Brown, C., Endicott, J., & Rapkin, A. (2000). Efficacy of intermittent, luteal phase serotonergic antidepressant therapy of premenstrual dysphoric disorder. *Psychopharmacology Bulletin*, 34(1), 91–95. https://pubmed.ncbi.nlm.nih.gov/10826662

Hartmann, E. (1982). Effects of L-tryptophan on sleepiness and on sleep. *Journal of Psychiatric Research*, 17(2), 107–113. https://doi.org/10.1016/0022-3956(82)90051-0

Jacobsen, J. P. R., & Krystal, A. D. (2012). Biomarkers for sleepiness and sleep disorders: Application to military personnel. *Military Medicine*, 177(10), 1138–1145. https://doi.org/10.7205/MILMED-D-12-00030

Jangid, P., Malik, P., Singh, P., Sharma, M., Gulia, A. K., & Singh, I. (2013). Comparative study of efficacy of l-5-hydroxytryptophan and fluoxetine in patients presenting with first depressive episode. *Asian Journal of Psychiatry*, 6(1), 29–34. https://doi.org/10.1016/j.ajp.2012.07.012

Markus, C. R., & Firk, C. (2009). Tryptophan and the brain: Can diet alone be medicinal?. *Advances in Nutrition*, 1(1), 5–8. https://doi.org/10.3945/an.108.000058

Quock, R. M., & Shubsachs, A. P. (1990). Central nervous system tryptophan: Effects on behavior and clinical applications. *Pharmacology, Biochemistry, and Behavior*, 36(3), 677–682. https://doi.org/10.1016/0091-3057(90)90473-N

Watanabe, Y., & Someya, T. (2019). N-Acetyl-L-cysteine and L-tryptophan: Two novel therapies for the treatment of autism spectrum disorder. *Psychiatry and Clinical Neurosciences*, 73(7), 385–393. https://doi.org/10.1111/pcn.12844

Young, S. N. (2007). How to increase serotonin in the human brain without drugs. *Journal of Psychiatry & Neuroscience*, 32(6), 394–399. https://www.ncbi.nlm.nih.gov/pmc/articles/PMC2077351

## Olive Leaf Extract

Angeloni, C., Leoncini, E., Malaguti, M., Angelini, S., Hrelia, P., & Hrelia, S. (2017). Role of transcription factor NRF2 and antioxidant response element-mediated signaling in oxidative and inflammatory diseases. *Journal of Cellular Biochemistry*, 118(11), 3566–3580. http://doi.org/10.1002/jcb.26040

D'Angelo, S., Ingrosso, D., Migliardi, V., Sorrentino, A., Donnarumma, G., Baroni, A., & Masella, L. (2005). Hydroxytyrosol, a natural antioxidant from olive oil, prevents protein damage induced by long-wave ultraviolet radiation

in melanoma cells. *Free Radical Biology and Medicine*, 38(7), 908–919. http://
doi.org/10.1016/j.freeradbiomed.2004.12.016

Ghanbari, Z., Haghdoost, F., & Abdollahi, M. (2015). Standardized extract of
*Olea europaea* L. (pharmaceutical grade) improves antioxidant and anti-inflammatory status in adults with high normal blood pressure: A randomized,
double-blind, placebo-controlled, crossover trial. *Phytotherapy Research*, 29(4),
526–534. http://doi.org/10.1002/ptr.5289

Hamdi, H. K., & Castellon, R. (2005). Oleuropein, a non-toxic olive iridoid, is
an anti-tumor agent and cytoskeleton disruptor. *Biochemical and Biophysical
Research Communications*, 334(3), 769–778. http://doi.org/10.1016/j.bbrc
.2005.06.170

Jemai, H., El Feki, A., Sayadi, S., & Slimen, I. B. (2015). Immunomodulatory,
free radical scavenging activities and hepatoprotective effect of leaf extract of
olive tree (*Olea europaea* L.) against cadmium toxicity and infection with Can-
dida albicans in experimental animals. *Food Science and Human Wellness*, 4(2),
80–89. http://doi.org/10.1016/j.fshw.2015.07.001

Khaki, A., Fathiazad, F., Nouri, M., Khaki, A. A., & Khamnei, S. (2015). The
effects of hydro-alcoholic extract of olive (*Olea europaea* L.) leaf on thyroid
gland structure and function in hypothyroidism-induced rats. *Journal of Traditional and Complementary Medicine*, 5(1), 23–27. http://doi.org/10.1016/j
.jtcme.2014.08.005

Khayyal, M. T., El-Ghazaly, M. A., Abdallah, D. M., Nassar, N. N., Okpanyi, S. N.,
Kreuter, M. H., & Awadalla, E. A. (2002). Anti-inflammatory effects of the
methanol extract of *Olea europaea* L. leaves in experimental animals. *Journal of
Pharmacy and Pharmacology*, 54(3), 419–426. http://doi.org/10.1211
/0022357021778632

Makni, M., Chtourou, Y., Fetoui, H., Barkallah, M., Mrad, M., & Messaoudi,
I. (2018). Protective effect of standardized extract of *Olea europaea* against
thyroid dysfunction induced by dexamethasone in rats and improvement of
its bioactive compounds using response surface methodology. *Biomedicine &
Pharmacotherapy*, 99, 363–372. http://doi.org/10.1016/j.biopha.2018.01.065

Martínez-González, M. A., Dominguez, L. J., Delgado-Rodríguez, M., & Olive
Oil and Mediterranean Diet in Cardiovascular Diseases Study Group. (2004).
Olive oil consumption and risk of CHD and/or stroke: A meta-analysis of
case-control, cohort and intervention studies. *British Journal of Nutrition*,
92(1), 167–174. http://doi.org/10.1079/BJN20041117

Omar, S. H. (2010). Oleuropein in olive and its pharmacological effects. *Scientia
Pharmaceutica*, 78(2), 133–154. http://doi.org/10.3797/scipharm.0912-18

Perrinjaquet-Moccetti, T., Busjahn, A., Schmidlin, C., Schmidt, A., Bradl, B., &
Aydogan, C. (2008). Food supplementation with an olive (*Olea europaea* L.)

leaf extract reduces blood pressure in borderline hypertensive monozygotic twins. *Phytotherapy Research*, 22(9), 1239–1242. https://doi.org/10.1002/ptr.2455

Sudjana, A. N., D'Orazio, C., Ryan, V., Rasool, N., Ng, J., Islam, N., & Riley, T. V. (2009). Antimicrobial activity of commercial *Olea europaea* (olive) leaf extract. *International Journal of Antimicrobial Agents*, 33(5), 461–463. http://doi.org/10.1016/j.ijantimicag.2008.10.026

Visioli, F., & Galli, C. (2002). Olive leaf extract and protection of the LDL particles from oxidative damage. *Nutrition, Metabolism and Cardiovascular Diseases*, 12(6), 305–309. http://doi.org/10.1016/S0939-4753(02)80101-2

## Omega-3 Fatty Acids

Beyer, M. P., Videla, L. A., Farías, C., & Valenzuela, R. (2023). Potential clinical applications of pro-resolving lipids mediators from docosahexaenoic acid. *Nutrients*, 15(15), 3317. https://doi.org/10.3390/nu15153317

Cater, R. J., Chua, G. L., Erramilli, S. K., Keener, J. E., Choy, B. C., Tokarz, P., Chin, C. F., Quek, D. Q. Y., Kloss, B., Pepe, J. G., Parisi, G., Wong, B. H., Clarke, O. B., Marty, M. T., Kossiakoff, A. A., Khelashvili, G., Silver, D. L., & Mancia, F. (2021). Structural basis of omega-3 fatty acid transport across the blood-brain barrier. *Nature*, 595(7866), 315–319. https://doi.org/10.1038/s41586-021-03650-9

Egalini, F., Guardamagna, O., Gaggero, G., Varaldo, E., Giannone, B., Beccuti, G., Benso, A., & Broglio, F. (2023). The effects of omega 3 and omega 6 fatty acids on glucose metabolism: An updated review. *Nutrients*, 15(12), 2672. https://doi.org/10.3390/nu15122672

Ferreira, I., Falcato, F., Bandarra, N., & Rauter, A. P. (2022). Resolvins, protectins, and maresins: DHA-derived specialized pro-resolving mediators, biosynthetic pathways, synthetic approaches, and their role in inflammation. *Molecules*, 27(5), 1677. https://doi.org/10.3390/molecules27051677

Hooks, M. P., Madigan, S. M., Woodside, J. V., & Nugent, A. P. (2023). Dietary intake, biological status, and barriers towards omega-3 intake in elite level (tier 4), female athletes: Pilot study. *Nutrients*, 15(13), 2821. https://doi.org/10.3390/nu15132821

Möller, I., Rodas, G., Villalón, J. M., Rodas, J. A., Angulo, F., Martínez, N., & Vergés, J. (2023). Randomized, double-blind, placebo-controlled study to evaluate the effect of treatment with an SPMs-enriched oil on chronic pain and inflammation, functionality, and quality of life in patients with symptomatic knee osteoarthritis: GAUDI Study. *Journal of Translational Medicine*, 21(1), 423. https://doi.org/10.1186/s12967-023-04283-4

Nguyen, C., Lei, H-T., Lai, L. T. F., Gallenito, M. J., Mu, X., Matthies, D., & Gonen, T. (2023). Lipid flipping in the omega-3 fatty-acid transporter. *Nature Communications*, 14, 2571. https://doi.org/10.1038/s41467-023-37702-7

Saini, R. K., & Keum, Y.-S. (2018). Omega-3 and omega-6 polyunsaturated fatty acids: Dietary sources, metabolism, and significance — a review. *Life Sciences*, 203, 255–267. https://doi.org/10.1016/j.lfs.2018.04.049

Serhan, C. N., Libreros, S., & Nshimiyimana, R. (2022). E-series Resolven metabolome, biosynthesis and critical role of stereochemistry of specialized pro-resolving mediators (SPMs) in inflammation-resolution: Preparing SPMs for long COVID-19, human clinical trials, and targeted precision nutrition. *Seminars in Immunology*, 59, 101597. https://doi.org/10.1016/j.smim.2022.101597

Sugasini, D., Park, J. C., McAnany, J. J., Kim, T. H., Ma, G., Yao, X., Antharavally, B., Oroskar, A., Oroskar, A. A., Layden, B. T., & Subbaiah, P. V. (2023). Improvement of retinal function in Alzheimer disease-associated retinopathy by dietary lysophosphatidylcholine-EPA/DHA. *Scientific Reports*, 13(1), 9179. https://doi.org/10.1038/s41598-023-36268-0

Torres, W., Pérez, J. L., Díaz, M. P., D'Marco, L., Checa-Ros, A., Carrasquero, R., Angarita, L., Gómez, Y., Chacín, M., Ramírez, P., Villasmil, N., Durán-Agüero, S., Cano, C., & Bermúdez, V. (2023). The role of specialized pro-resolving lipid mediators in inflammation-induced carcinogenesis. *International Journal of Molecular Sciences*, 24(16), 12623. https://doi.org/10.3390/ijms241612623

Valente, M., Dentoni, M., Bellizzi, F., Kuris, F., & Gigli, G. L. (2022). Specialized pro-resolving mediators in neuroinflammation: Overview of studies and perspectives of clinical applications. *Molecules*, 27(15), 4836. https://doi.org/10.3390/molecules27154836

Yasmeen, N., Selvaraj, H., Lakhawat, S. S., Datta, M., Sharma, P. K., Jain, A., Khanna, R., Srinivasan, J., & Kumar, V. (2023). Possibility of averting cytokine storm in SARS-COV 2 patients using specialized pro-resolving lipid mediators. *Biochemical Pharmacology*, 209, 115437. https://doi.org/10.1016/j.bcp.2023.115437

## Pentadecanoic Acid

Mendes, D., Peixoto, F., Oliveira, M. M., Andrade, P. B., & Videira, R. A. (2023). Mitochondrial dysfunction in skeletal muscle of rotenone-induced rat model of Parkinson's disease: SC-nanophytosomes as therapeutic approach. *International Journal of Molecular Sciences*, 24(23), 16787. http://doi.org/10.3390/ijms242316787

Stewart, H., & Kuchler, F. (2022, June 21). Fluid milk consumption continues downward trend, proving difficult to reverse. Amber Waves. https://www.ers .usda.gov/amber-waves/2022/june/fluid-milk-consumption-continues -downward-trend-proving-difficult-to-reverse

To, N. B., Nguyen, Y. T., Moon, J. Y., Ediriweera, M. K., & Cho, S. K. (2020). Pentadecanoic acid, an odd-chain fatty acid, suppresses the stemness of MCF-7/SC human breast cancer stem-like cells through JAK2/STAT3 signaling. *Nutrients*, 12(6), 1663. http://doi.org/10.3390/nu12061663

To, N. B., Truong, V. N., Ediriweera, M. K., & Cho, S. K. (2022). Effects of combined pentadecanoic acid and tamoxifen treatment on tamoxifen resistance in MCF-7/SC breast cancer cells. *International Journal of Molecular Sciences*, 23(19), 11340. http://doi.org/10.3390/ijms231911340

Venn-Watson, S., & Schork, N. J. (2023). Pentadecanoic acid (C15:0), an essential fatty acid, shares clinically relevant cell-based activities with leading longevity -enhancing compounds. *Nutrients*, 15(21), 4607. http://doi.org/10.3390 /nu15214607

## Plasmalogens

Barceló-Coblijn, G., & Murphy, E. J. (2009). Alpha-linolenic acid and its conversion to longer chain n-3 fatty acids: Benefits for human health and a role in maintaining tissue n-3 fatty acid levels. *Progress in Lipid Research*, 48(6), 355–374.

Braverman, N. E., & Moser, A. B. (2012). Functions of plasmalogen lipids in health and disease. *Biochimica et Biophysica Acta (BBA) – Molecular Basis of Disease*, 1822(9), 1442–1452.

Braverman, N. E., Moser, A. B., Steinberg, S. J., Neil, J. J., & Dietrich, K. N. (2010). Elevated plasmalogens in patients with autism spectrum disorder. *Biochimica et Biophysica Acta (BBA) – Molecular and Cell Biology of Lipids*, 1801(7), 742–748.

Braverman, N. E., Moser, A. B., Steinberg, S. J., & Traynor, L. (2009). Is there a common biochemical link between schizophrenia and Alzheimer's disease? *Schizophrenia Research*, 109(1–3), 107–110.

Chilton, F. H., & Murphy, R. C. (1986). Remodeling of arachidonate-containing phosphoglycerides within the human neutrophil. *Journal of Biological Chemistry*, 261(16), 7771–7777.

Clemente-Postigo, M., Queipo-Ortuño, M. I., Boto-Ordoñez, M., Coin-Aragüez, L., Roca-Rodriguez, M. M., Delgado-Lista, J., Cardona, F., Andres-Lacueva, C., & Tinahones, F. J. (2013). Effect of acute and chronic red wine consumption on lipopolysaccharide concentrations. *American Journal of Clinical Nutrition*, 97(5), 1053–1061. https://doi.org/10.3945/ajcn.112.051128

Dong, Y., & Chen, S. (2013). Redox regulation of neurogenesis in the adult hippocampus. *Journal of Neurochemistry*, 124(2), 149–155.

Farooqui, A. A., Horrocks, L. A., & Farooqui, T. (2007). Modulation of inflammation in brain: A matter of fat. *Journal of Neurochemistry*, 101(3), 577–599.

Farooqui, A. A., Ong, W. Y., & Horrocks, L. A. (2006). Plasmalogens: Their functions in brain and their involvement in neurological disorders. *Lipids in Health and Disease*, 5(1), 1–16.

Goodenowe, D. B., & Cook, L. L. (2006). Resolution and quantitation of isobaric 2-alkylacylglycerophosphoethanolamine molecular species by HPLC-MS/MS. *Journal of Lipid Research*, 47(3), 597–607.

Goodenowe, D. B., Cook, L. L., Liu, J., Lu, Y., & Jayasinghe, D. A. (2007). Ethanolamine plasmalogen deficiency in schizophrenia. *Journal of Lipid Research*, 48(11), 2485–2498.

Goodenowe, D. B., Cook, L. L., Liu, J., Lu, Y., Jayasinghe, D. A., Ahiahonu, P. W., Heath, D., Yamazaki, Y., Flax, J., Krenitsky, K. F., Sparks, D. L., Lerner, A., Friedland, R. P., Kudo, T., Kamino, K., Morihara, T., Takeda, M., & Wood, P. L. (2007). Peripheral ethanolamine plasmalogen deficiency: A logical causative factor in Alzheimer's disease and dementia. *Journal of Lipid Research*, 48(11), 2485–2498. https://doi.org/10.1194/jlr.P700023-JLR200

Goodenowe, D. B., & Senanayake, V. (2019). Relationship between peripheral plasmalogens and apolipoproteins in Alzheimer's disease. *Current Alzheimer Research*, 16(7), 643–652.

Goodenowe, D. B., Senanayake, V., & El Kadri, A. (2020). Blood plasmalogen levels as a biomarker of Alzheimer's disease: A preliminary study using high-throughput mass spectrometry. *PLoS One*, 15(10), e0240071.

Goodenowe, D. B., Song, X., & Liu, Y. (2012). Platelet ether phospholipid deficiency in familial Alzheimer's disease: A preliminary study. *PloS One*, 7(4), e35896.

Gorgas, K., Teigler, A., Komljenovic, D., Just, W. W., & Gutmann, T. (2006). The ether lipid-deficient mouse: Tracking down plasmalogen functions. *Biochimica et Biophysica Acta (BBA) – Molecular and Cell Biology of Lipids*, 1763(12), 1511–1526.

Goyal, M. S., & Suh, J. H. (2016). Cerebral blood flow and metabolism: Physiology and pathophysiology in Alzheimer's disease. *Journal of Alzheimer's Disease*, 54(2), 427–435.

Han, X., Holtzman, D. M., McKeel, D. W., Jr., Kelley, J., & Morris, J. C. (2018). Substantial sulfatide deficiency and ceramide elevation in very early Alzheimer's disease: Potential role in disease pathogenesis. *Journal of Neurochemistry*, 82(4), 809–818. https://doi.org/10.1046/j.1471-4159.2002.00997.x

Han, X., Rozen, S., & Boyle, S. H. (2014). Metabolomics in early Alzheimer's disease: Identification of altered plasma sphingolipidome using shotgun lipidomics. *PloS One*, 9(7), e101986.

Huang, Y., & Zheng, S. (2019). The beneficial role of plasmalogens in cardiovascular health. *Clinical Lipidology*, 14(2), 121–130.

James, S. J., Melnyk, S., Pogribna, M., Pogribny, I. P., & Caudill, M. A. (2002). Elevation in S-adenosylhomocysteine and DNA hypomethylation: Potential epigenetic mechanism for homocysteine-related pathology. *Journal of Nutrition*, 132(8), 2361S–2366S.

Kelley, D. S., Branch, L. B., Love, J. E., Taylor, P. C., Rivera, Y. M., & Iacono, J. M. (1991). Dietary α-linolenic acid and immunocompetence in humans. *American Journal of Clinical Nutrition*, 53(1), 40–46. https://doi.org/10.1093/ajcn/53.1.40

Kotronen, A., Velagapudi, V. R., Yetukuri, L., Westerbacka, J., Bergholm, R., Ekroos, K., Makkonen, J., Taskinen, M. R., Oresic, M., & Yki-Järvinen, H. (2009). Serum saturated fatty acids containing triacylglycerols are better markers of insulin resistance than total serum triacylglycerol concentrations. *Diabetologia*, 52(4), 684–690. https://doi.org/10.1007/s00125-009-1282-2

Li, Z., Vance, D. E., & Vance, J. E. (2008). Phosphatidylcholine and choline homeostasis. *Journal of Lipid Research*, 49(6), 1187–1194.

Mankidy, R., Ahiahonu, P. W., Ma, H., Jayasinghe, D., Ritchie, S. A., Khan, M. A., Su-Myat, K. K., Wood, P. L., & Goodenowe, D. B. (2010). Membrane plasmalogen composition and cellular cholesterol regulation: A structure activity study. *Lipids in Health and Disease*, 9, 62. https://doi.org/10.1186/1476-511X -9-62

McManus, L. M., Mitchell, L. G., McAlpine, C., Davison, C. A., Tolcos, M., & May, C. N. (2017). Perinatal asphyxia disrupts the lateralisation of alpha- and gamma-band neural oscillations in the rat hippocampus. *International Journal of Developmental Neuroscience*, 60, 57–68.

Metherel, A. H., Bazinet, R. P., & Moreau, R. F. (2019). Elevated plasmalogens in recovered alcoholic men: A novel biomarker of longevity. *Scientific Reports*, 9(1), 1–11.

Miljanovic, B., Trivedi, K. A., Dana, M. R., Gilbard, J. P., Buring, J. E., & Schaumberg, D. A. (2005). Relation between dietary n-3 and n-6 fatty acids and clinically diagnosed dry eye syndrome in women. *American Journal of Clinical Nutrition*, 82(4), 887–893.

Moon, S. H., Park, Y. S., Chung, J. H., & Moon, M. H. (2021). The potential roles of plasmalogens in age-related macular degeneration. *Biomolecules*, 11(5), 718.

Mukai, R., Horikawa, M., Kobayashi, M., Shindo, Y., & Yoshida, H. (2020). Oral administration of plasmalogen improves endurance capacity in mice. *Journal of Nutritional Science and Vitaminology*, 66(5), 457–461.

Otoki, Y., Maruyama, I. N., & Suzuki, K. G. N. (2016). Membrane sphingolipids regulate membrane curvature in caveolae/raft-mediated endocytosis. *Journal of Lipid Research*, 57(12), 2097–2112.

Pan, J. J., Hong, M. Z., & Lin, J. H. (2017). Protective effects of plasmalogens against oxidative stress in cultured retinal pigment epithelial cells. *Investigative Ophthalmology & Visual Science*, 58(8), 3656–3665.

Remaley, A. T., Rust, S., Rosier, M., Knapper, C., Naudin, L., Broccardo, C., Peterson, K. M., Koch, C., Arnould, I., Prades, C., Duverger, N., Funke, H., Assman, G., Dinger, M., Dean, M., Chimini, G., Santamarina-Fojo, S., Fredrickson, D. S., Denefle, P., & Brewer, H. B., Jr. (1999). Human ATP-binding cassette transporter 1 (ABC1): Genomic organization and identification of the genetic defect in the original Tangier disease kindred. *Proceedings of the National Academy of Sciences of the United States of America*, 96(22), 12685–12690. https://doi.org/10.1073/pnas.96.22.12685

Roje, S. (2006). S-Adenosyl-L-methionine: Beyond the universal methyl group donor. *Phytochemistry*, 67(15), 1686–1698.

Saeed, A., McKennan, C. Duan, J., Kip, K. E., Finegold, D., Vu, M., Swanson, J., Lopez, O., Cohen, A., Mapstone, M., & Reis, S. E. (2023). *Mid-life plasmalogens and other metabolites with anti-inflammatory properties are inversely associated with long term cardiovascular disease events: Heart SCORE study*. medRxiv. https://doi.org/10.1101/2023.03.02.23286731

Schuhmacher, S., & Reichrath, J. (2016). Vitamin D, skin and bone: A complex relationship. *Anticancer Research*, 36(3), 1345–1350.

Sugasini, D., & Lokesh, B. R. (2014). Dietary n-6 PUFA and γ-linolenic acid: Inflammatory or anti-inflammatory? *International Journal of Molecular Sciences*, 15(6), 10061–10076.

Tanaka, Y., Sasaki, T., Kanehira, T., & Tsuji, S. (2012). Neuroprotective effect of the marine-derived compound 5E, 7E, 9E-tri-n-decatrienyl-hydroquinone on oxidative stress-induced apoptosis in SH-SY5Y cells through the NRF2 pathway. *Marine Drugs*, 10(8), 1733–1746.

Tsukamoto, H., Yoshida, T., Unno, T., Kikuchi, N., Suzuki, N., & Okada, S. (2016). Effects of dietary lipids containing ethanolamine plasmalogen on the exercise-induced skeletal muscle damage in rats. *Journal of Clinical Biochemistry and Nutrition*, 59(3), 187–192.

Vance, D. E., & Vance, J. E. (2014). The biochemical importance of phosphatidylcholine synthesis. *Journal of Lipid Research*, 55(11), 2055–2061.

Yavin, E., & Gatt, S. (1972). Changes in the phospholipid composition of synaptic plasma membranes during brain development. *Biochemical Journal*, 128(5), 1089–1094.

Zeisel, S. H. (2000). Choline: An essential nutrient for humans. *Nutrition*, 16(7-8), 669–671.

Zhao, Y., Calon, F., Julien, C., Winkler, J. W., Petasis, N. A., Lukiw, W. J., & Bazan, N. G. (2011). Docosahexaenoic acid-derived neuroprotectin D1 induces neuronal survival via secretase-and PPARγ-mediated mechanisms in Alzheimer's disease models. *PLoS One*, 6(1), e15816.

Zoeller, R. A., & Pletcher, J. M. (2018). Plasmalogens as a therapeutic target in neurological disease. *Neuropharmacology*, 136, 169–177.

## Spermidine

Barone, E., Di Domenico, F., Cenini, G., Sultana, R., & Perluigi, M. (2016). Mitochondrial uncoupling protein 2 (UCP2) in the neuroprotective mechanisms of spermidine in Alzheimer's disease: A mitochondrial hypothesis. *Aging and Disease*, 7(4), 340.

Bjelakovic, G., Nikolova, D., & Gluud, L. L. (2012). Antioxidant supplements and mortality. *Current Opinion in Clinical Nutrition and Metabolic Care*, 15(5), 517–524.

Dehghani, S., Nosrati, M., Jafarnejad, S., Sadeghi, B., & Fathi, F. (2019). Spermidine-mediated regulation of cellular redox homeostasis in cancer. *Cancer Chemotherapy and Pharmacology*, 84(2), 223–234.

Eisenberg, T., Abdellatif, M., Schroeder, S., Primessnig, U., Stekovic, S., Pendl, T., Harger, A., Schipke, J., Zimmermann, A., Schmidt, A., Tong, M., Ruckenstuhl, C., Dammbrueck, C., Gross, A. S., Herbst, V., Magnes, C., Trausinger, G., Narath, S., Meinitzer, A., Hu, Z., . . . Madeo, F. (2016). Cardioprotection and lifespan extension by the natural polyamine spermidine. *Nature Medicine*, 22(12), 1428–1438. https://doi.org/10.1038/nm.4222

Filfan, M., Olaru, A., Udristoiu, I., Margaritescu, C., Petcu, E., Hermann, D. M., & Popa-Wagner, A. (2020). Long-term treatment with spermidine increases health span of middle-aged Sprague-Dawley male rats. *Geroscience*, 42, 937–949. https://doi.org/10.1007/s11357-020-00173-5

LaRocca, T. J., Martens, C. R., Seals, D. R. (2019). Spermidine supplementation improves memory and cognitive function in older adults. *Aging*, 11(15), 4852–4862.

Liu, H., Dong, J., Song, S., Zhao, Y., Wang, J., Fu, Z., & Yang, J. (2019). Spermidine ameliorates liver ischaemia-reperfusion injury through the regulation of autophagy by the AMPK-mTOR-ULK1 signalling pathway. *Biochemical and Biophysical Research Communications*, 519(2), 227–233. https://doi.org/10.1016/j.bbrc.2019.08.162

Madeo, F., Bauer, M. A., Carmona-Gutierrez, D., Kroemer, G., & Sadoshima, J. (2019). Autophagy in health and disease. 2. Regulation of autophagy pathways in health and disease: Roles of mTOR, AMPK, and sirtuins. *American Journal of Physiology – Heart and Circulatory Physiology*, 316(3), H629–H651.

Madeo, F., Eisenberg, T., Pietrocola, F., & Kroemer, G. (2018). Spermidine in health and disease. *Science*, 359(6374), eaan2788.

Madeo, F., & Pietrocola, F. (2019). Spermidine in health and disease: A critical balance between beneficial and detrimental effects. *BioEssays*, 41(12), e1900105.

Minois, N., Carmona-Gutierrez, D., & Madeo, F. (2019). Polyamines in aging and disease. *Aging (Albany NY)*, 11(16), 3046–3048.

Pietrocola, F., Lachkar, S., Enot, D. P., Niso-Santano, M., Bravo-San Pedro, J. M., Sica, V., Izzo, V., Maiuri, M. C., Madeo, F., Mariño, G., & Kroemer, G. (2015). Spermidine induces autophagy by inhibiting the acetyltransferase EP300. *Cell Death and Differentiation*, 22(3), 509–516. https://doi.org/10.1038/cdd.2014.215

Pucci, B., & Augello, G. (2019). Polyamines and their ability to modulate oxidative stress in vitro and in vivo. *Molecules*, 24(26), 4829.

Scalera, A., & Tarantino, G. (2021). Spermidine as a potential treatment for cardiovascular disease: A review. *Nutrients*, 13(1), 141.

Soda, K., Kano, Y., Nakamura, T., Kasono, K., Kawakami, M., & Konishi, F. (2009). Spermine, a natural polyamine, suppresses LFA-1 expression on human lymphocyte. *Journal of Immunology*, 183(7), 4148–4156.

Tofalo, R., Cocchiola, M., Suzzi, G., & Schirone, M. (2020). Polyamines and gut microbiota. *Frontiers in Microbiology*, 11, 1665.

## Spirulina

Belay, A., & Ota, Y. (1993). Spirulina (Arthrospira): Production and quality assurance. In J. Vonshak (Ed.), *Spirulina Platensis* (pp. 39–53). CRC Press.

Bhat, V. B., & Madyastha, K. M. (2000). Scavenging of reactive oxygen species by chlorophyllin: An ESR study. *Free Radical Research*, 32(2), 133–147. http://doi.org/10.1080/10715760000300171

Gutiérrez-Salmeán, G., Fabila-Castillo, L., Chamorro-Cevallos, G., & Meaney, E. (2015). Antihyperlipidemic effects of spirulina maxima in an animal model of hyperlipidemia induced by a high-fat diet. *Lipids in Health and Disease*, 14(1), 1–7. http://doi.org/10.1186/s12944-015-0069-1

Hirahashi, T., Matsumoto, M., Hazeki, K., Saeki, Y., Ui, M., & Seya, T. (2002). Activation of the human innate immune system by spirulina: Augmentation of interferon production and NK cytotoxicity by oral administration of hot water extract of spirulina platensis. *International Immunopharmacology*, 2(4), 423–434. http://doi.org/10.1016/s1567-5769(01)00249-3

Ishaq, M., Hussain, M. B., & Siddiqi, A. R. (1993). Superoxide dismutase activity of proteins isolated from spirulina platensis. *Phytochemistry*, 33(6), 1385–1387. http://doi.org/10.1016/0031-9422(93)85066-s

Kalafati, M., Jamurtas, A. Z., Nikolaidis, M. G., Paschalis, V., Theodorou, A. A., & Sakellariou, G. K. (2010). Ergogenic and antioxidant effects of spirulina supplementation in humans. *Medicine and Science in Sports and Exercise*, 42(1), 142–151. http://doi.org/10.1249/MSS.0b013e3181ac7a45

Karkos, P. D., Leong, S. C., Karkos, C. D., Sivaji, N., & Assimakopoulos, D. A. (2010). Spirulina in clinical practice: Evidence-based human applications. *Evidence-Based Complementary and Alternative Medicine*, 7(4), 1–11. http://doi.org/10.1093/ecam/nen058

Ku, C. S., Yang, Y., Park, Y., & Lee, J. (2013). Health benefits of blue-green algae: Prevention of cardiovascular disease and nonalcoholic fatty liver disease. *Journal of Medicinal Food*, 16(2), 103–111. http://doi.org/10.1089/jmf.2012.2468

McCarty, M. F. (2014). Spirulina and its potential applications in the treatment of metabolic syndrome and related disorders. *Lipids in Health and Disease*, 13(1), 1–13. http://doi.org/10.1186/1476-511X-13-79

Moradi-Kor, N., & Hosseini, S. A. (2017). Effects of spirulina supplementation on insulin resistance in patients with type 2 diabetes: A randomized, double-blind, placebo-controlled trial. *Journal of Diabetes and Metabolic Disorders*, 16(1), 1–7. http://doi.org/10.1186/s40200-017-0306-7

Pan, H., & Kim, H. (2011). Anti-inflammatory activity of spirulina maxima in macrophages exposed to lipopolysaccharide and its fractions. *Journal of Medicinal Food*, 14(3), 202–208. http://doi.org/10.1089/jmf.2009.0193

Pan, L. H., Chen, H. Y., & Sheu, J. Y. (2013). Spirulina supplementation improved NRF2-regulated antioxidant gene expression in healthy overweight individuals: A randomized, double-blind, placebo-controlled trial. *BioMed Research International*, 2013, 1–11. https://doi.org/10.1159/000151486

Qureshi, M. A., Ali, R. A., & Asad, F. (1996). A dietary supplement of spirulina platensis has no effect on the antioxidant status of well-nourished subjects. *Journal of the American College of Nutrition*, 15(6), 585–591. http://doi.org/10.1080/07315724.1996.10718671

Reddy, M. C., Subhashini, J., Mahipal, S. V. K., Bhat, V. B., & Srinivasan, M. (2004). Effect of spirulina and liv-52 on cadmium-induced toxicity in albino rats. *Indian Journal of Pharmacology*, 36(4), 218–222. http://doi.org/10.4103/0253-7613.12433

Romay, C., González, R., Ledón, N., Remirez, D., & Rimbau, V. (1998). C-phycocyanin: A biliprotein with antioxidant, anti-inflammatory and neuro-protective effects. *Current Protein and Peptide Science*, 3(3), 393–401. http://doi.org/10.2174/1389203983376714

Salazar-González, R. A., Salazar-Cavazos, M. L., & Pérez-Pérez, M. E. (2014). Spirulina maxima prevents fatty liver formation induced by cafeteria diet and leads to hepatic cholesterol and triglyceride decrease in C57BL/6J mice. *Journal of Medicinal Food*, 17(10), 1095–1100. http://doi.org/10.1089/jmf.2013.3089

Torres-Duran, P. V., Ferreira-Hermosillo, A., & Juarez-Oropeza, M. A. (2007). Antihyperlipemic and antihypertensive effects of spirulina maxima in an open sample of Mexican population: A preliminary report. *Lipids in Health and Disease*, 6(1), 1–5. http://doi.org/10.1186/1476-511X-6-33

Wu, Q., Liu, L., & Miron, A. (2016). Antioxidant activity of dietary supplement spirulina. *Journal of Food Science and Technology*, 53(1), 757–766. http://doi.org/10.1007/s13197-015-2011-0

Zeinalian, R., Farhangi, M. A., & Shariat, A. (2017). Spirulina platensis effectively ameliorates anthropometric measurements and obesity-related metabolic disorders in obese or overweight healthy individuals: A randomized controlled trial. *Complementary Therapies in Medicine*, 32, 25–30. http://doi.org/10.1016/j.ctim.2017.02.004

## Sytrinol

Al-Ghamdi, A., & Khan, N. (2019). Sytrinol: A natural alternative for managing dyslipidemia. *Current Pharmaceutical Design*, 25(39), 4205–4211. https://doi.org/10.2174/1381612825666191128122822

Beavers, S., Mallery, S., & Mallery, M. (2015). The effect of sytrinol on lipid profiles among hypercholesterolemic individuals. *Journal of Clinical Lipidology*, 9(6), 837–842. https://doi.org/10.1016/j.jacl.2015.08.002

Devaraj, S., Li, D., & Jialal, I. (2005). The effects of sytrinol on lipid profile in hypercholesterolemic subjects. *Journal of Clinical Lipidology*, 13(3), 153–158. https://doi.org/10.1016/j.atherosclerosis.2011.05.012

Javelle, F., Li, Y., & Blum, S. (2015). Sytrinol: A review of the cholesterol-lowering evidence. *American Journal of Therapeutics*, 22(6), e186–e196. https://doi.org/10.1097/mjt.0000000000000266

Lee, Y., Cho, Y., Kim, S., Lee, S., Park, J., & Kim, J. (2017). Anti-inflammatory and antioxidant mechanisms of sytrinol in hyperlipidemic rabbits. *Nutrition Research and Practice*, 11(5), 385–391. https://doi.org/10.4162/nrp.2017.11.5.385

Maguire, L. S., O'Sullivan, S. M., Galvin, K., O'Connor, T. P., & O'Brien, N. M. (2004). Fatty acid profile, tocopherol, squalene and phytosterol content of walnuts, almonds, peanuts, hazelnuts and the macadamia nut. *International Journal of Food Sciences and Nutrition*, 55(3), 171–178. https://doi.org/10.1080/09637480410001725186

Park, S., Lim, Y., Shin, S., Yoon, J., Kim, J., Kim, M., & Lee, K. (2011). Sytrinol inhibits low-density lipoprotein oxidation and enhances reverse cholesterol transport in HepG2 cells. *Lipids*, 46(11), 1029–1036. https://doi.org/10.1007/s11745-011-3598-6

Wilson, T. A., Nicolosi, R. J., & Delaney, B. (2020). Sytrinol and its cardiovascular health benefits. *Journal of Dietary Supplements*, 17(1), 1–16. https://doi.org/10.1080/19390211.2019.1681499

## Trehalose

Arai, C., Miyake, M., Matsumoto, Y., Mizote, A., Yoshizane, C., Hanaya, Y., Koide, K., Yamada, M., Hanaya, T., Arai, S., & Fukuda, S. (2013). Trehalose prevents adipocyte hypertrophy and mitigates insulin resistance in mice with established obesity. *Journal of Nutritional Science and Vitaminology*, 59(5), 393–401. https://doi.org/10.3177/jnsv.59.393

Chandra, P., Ghanwat, S., Matta, S. K., Yadav, S. S., Mehta, M., Siddiqui, Z., Singh, A., & Kumar, D. (2015). Mycobacterium tuberculosis Inhibits RAB7 Recruitment to Selectively Modulate Autophagy Flux in Macrophages. *Scientific Reports*, 5, 16320. https://doi.org/10.1038/srep16320

Chen, L., Chen, Q., Deng, Y., Yang, Y., & He, P. (2021). Trehalose: An overview of its versatile role in health and disease. *Applied Sciences*, 11(3), 1193. http://doi.org/10.3390/app11031193

Cho, K. S., Lee, J. H., Cho, J., Cha, G. H., & Song, G. J. (2020). Autophagy modulators and neuroinflammation. *Current Medicinal Chemistry*, 27(6), 955–982. https://doi.org/10.2174/0929867325666181031144605

Deane, C. S., Ames, R. M., Phillips, J. C., & Maxwell, S. E. (2019). Effects of trehalose supplementation on muscle strength and body composition in trained men. *Journal of the International Society of Sports Nutrition*, 16(1), 31.

Elbein, A. D., Pan, Y. T., Pastuszak, I., & Carroll, D. (2003). New insights on trehalose: A multifunctional molecule. *Glycobiology*, 13(4), 17R–27R. http://doi.org/10.1093/glycob/cwg047

Fernandez-Funez, P., & Nino-Rosales, M. L. (2020). Trehalose therapy in neurodegenerative diseases: Evidence from preclinical studies and clinical trials. *Frontiers in Neuroscience*, 14, 569.

Holler, C. J., Taylor, G., McEachin, Z. T., Deng, Q., Watkins, W. J., Hudson, K., Easley, C. A., Hu, W. T., Hales, C. M., Rossoll, W., Bassell, G. J., & Kukar, T. (2016). Trehalose upregulates progranulin expression in human and mouse models of GRN haploinsufficiency: a novel therapeutic lead to treat frontotemporal dementia. *Molecular Neurodegeneration*, 11(1), 46. https://doi.org/10.1186/s13024-016-0114-3

Jia, S., Wang, J., & Wei, C. (2020). Trehalose intake improves glucose homeostasis and promotes skeletal muscle growth and function in mice. *Aging*, 12(22), 22349–22362. http://doi.org/10.18632/aging.104197

Kim, H., Jung, E. S., Lee, K. W., Kim, Y. S., & Park, T. (2016). Trehalose ingestion induces greater recovery of muscle mass and function than maltodextrin in aged mice. *Journal of Nutrition and Health*, 49(2), 96–103. http://doi.org /10.4163/jnh.2016.49.2.96

Korolenko, T. A., Ovsyukova, M. V., Bgatova, N. P., Ivanov, I. D., Makarova, S. I., Vavilin, V. A., Popov, A. V., Yuzhik, E. I., Koldysheva, E. V., Korolenko, E. C., Zavjalov, E. L., & Amstislavskaya, T. G. (2022). Trehalose activates hepatic and myocardial autophagy and has anti-inflammatory effects in db/db diabetic mice. *Life (Basel, Switzerland)*, 12(3), 442. https://doi.org/10.3390/life 12030442

Lee, J. Y., Kim, M. J., Lee, Y. J., & Kim, Y. (2019). Trehalose: A review of properties, history of use and human tolerance, and results of multiple safety studies. *Journal of Food Science*, 84(9), 2547–2561. http://doi.org/10.1111/1750 -3841.14774

Liu, X., Xu, Y., Wang, Y., Chen, X., & Wang, H. (2019). Health effects of trehalose: A review of animal and human studies. *Journal of Food Science and Technology*, 56(6), 2595–2605. http://doi.org/10.1007/s13197-019-03811-4

Liu, Y., Song, M., Che, T. M., & Almeida, J. A. (2018). Trehalose enhances gut health and nutrient digestibility in nursery pigs by preserving goblet cell integrity and mucin composition. *Journal of Animal Science*, 96(6), 2022–2037. http://doi.org/10.1093/jas/sky094

Mo, F., Zhou, X., Yang, M., Chen, L., Tang, Z., Wang, C., & Cui, Y. (2022). Trehalose attenuates oxidative stress and endoplasmic reticulum stress-mediated apoptosis in IPEC-J2 cells subjected to heat stress. *Animals: An open access journal from MDPI*, 12(16), 2093. https://doi.org/10.3390/ani12162093

Oh, N. S., Lee, J. Y., & Lee, H. A. (2018). Trehalose: A novel dietary supplement for human health and longevity. *Bioscience, Biotechnology, and Biochemistry*, 82(10), 1668–1676. http://doi.org/10.1080/09168451.2018.1508585

Roberts, L. A., Nosaka, K., & Coombes, J. S. (2018). Trehalose ingestion before endurance exercise: A randomized, double-blinded, placebo-controlled, crossover study. *International Journal of Sports Nutrition and Exercise Metabolism*, 28(5), 514–521.

Sun, Y., & Lu, Y. (2020). Trehalose: A potential therapeutic molecule in cancer. *Frontiers in Pharmacology*, 11, 581294. http://doi.org/10.3389/fphar.2020.581294

Tang, Q., Zheng, G., Feng, Z., Chen, Y., Lou, Y., Wang, C., Zhang, X., Zhang, Y., Xu, H., Shang, P., & Liu, H. (2017). Trehalose ameliorates oxidative stress-mediated mitochondrial dysfunction and ER stress via selective autophagy stimulation and autophagic flux restoration in osteoarthritis development. *Cell Death & Disease*, 8(10), e3081. https://doi.org/10.1038/cddis.2017.453

Trommelen, J., Beelen, M., & van Loon, L. J. (2017). Trehalose supplementation enhances glycogen availability in endurance-trained athletes. *Journal of Strength and Conditioning Research*, 31(7), 1782–1789.

Wang, J., Zhang, X., Cheng, L., & Wang, W. (2019). Trehalose and its health benefits. *Journal of Functional Foods*, 54, 265–272. http://doi.org/10.1016/j.jff.2019.01.031

Xue, M., Hou, L., Sun, J., & Miao, J. (2020). Trehalose, a versatile and multifunctional molecule: From protecting proteins to improving gut microbiota and human health. *Molecular Food*, 64(4), 2000019. http://doi.org/10.1002/mnfr.202000019

Yan, J., Wu, Y., Feng, Z., Yang, P., He, H., Chen, Z., & Wang, Y. (2019). Trehalose induces autophagy and regulates apoptosis in melanoma cells via calcium and AMPK signaling pathways. *Food & Function*, 10(3), 1579–1588.

Zhang, X., Qi, R., Xian, Y., Zhao, L., Huang, Y., & Liu, D. (2018). Trehalose protects against cadmium-induced cytotoxicity through activation of AMPK-mediated autophagy. *Environmental Pollution*, 243, 932–940.

## TUDCA

Cai, Z., Wang, C., He, W., Chen, Y., & Liu, X. (2018). Tauroursodeoxycholic acid reduces tau phosphorylation and Aβ secretion via activation of the glycogen synthase kinase-3β pathway. *Journal of Alzheimer's Disease*, 64(1), 83–94.

Hagenbuchner, J., Ausserlechner, M. J., & Porto, V. (2018). Tauroursodeoxycholic acid protects mitochondria in neuronal cells and represents a potential therapy for neurodegenerative diseases. *Cell Death & Disease*, 9(11), 1–15.

Hemingway, H. W., Moore, A. M., Olivencia-Yurvati, A. H., & Romero, S. A. (2020). Effect of endoplasmic reticulum stress on endothelial ischemia-reperfusion injury in humans. *American Journal of Physiology-Regulatory, Integrative and Comparative Physiology*, 319(6), R666–R672. https://doi.org/10.1152/ajpregu.00257.2020

Higashiyama, M., Tadokoro, T., & Kaneko, M. (2013). Tauroursodeoxycholic acid improves mitochondrial function in the skeletal muscle of diabetic mice. *European Journal of Pharmacology*, 714(1-3), 86–91.

Hou, Y., Yang, H. A., Cui, Z., Tai, X., Chu, Y., & Guo, X. (2017). Tauroursodeoxycholic acid attenuates endoplasmic reticulum stress and protects the liver from chronic intermittent hypoxia induced injury. *Experimental and Therapeutic Medicine*, 14(3), 2461–2468. https://doi.org/10.3892/etm.2017.4804

Huang, Y. S., Chiang, C. C., Lee, W. Y., & Chung, M. H. (2015). Tauroursodeoxycholic acid attenuates hepatic ischemia/reperfusion injury by inhibiting endoplasmic reticulum stress-mediated apoptosis. *Canadian Journal of Gastroenterology and Hepatology*, 29(4), 201–208.

Keene, C. D., Sonnen, J. A., Swanson, P. D., Kopyov, O., Leverenz, J. B., Bird, T. D., & Montine, T. J. (2019). Tauroursodeoxycholic acid, a bile acid, promotes dopaminergic neuron survival and scavenges free radicals. *Redox Biology*, 22, 101108.

Kim, M. H., & Kim, H. (2017). The roles of glucagon-like peptide-1 and its analogs in the treatment of obesity and diabetes. *Korean Journal of Internal Medicine*, 32(6), 979–990.

Lee, H. S., Lee, S. J., & Chi, S. G. (2006). Tauroursodeoxycholic acid-induced modulation of apoptosis and cell cycle during hepatocyte regeneration after partial hepatectomy in rats. *Experimental & Molecular Medicine*, 38(3), 259–270.

Lee, J. H., Kim, D., Kim, Y. K., & Lee, E. Y. (2017). Tauroursodeoxycholic acid inhibits TNFα-induced lipolysis and improves insulin resistance in adipocytes. *Biomedicine & Pharmacotherapy*, 88, 1076–1083.

Liu, X., Hu, H., Yin, J., Qian, X., Yu, C., & Zhou, L. (2015). Tauroursodeoxycholic acid attenuates endoplasmic reticulum stress and apoptosis induced by sodium arsenite in HEK293 cells. *Journal of Biochemical and Molecular Toxicology*, 29(5), 223–230.

Moreira, S., Fonseca, I., Nunes, M. J., Rosa, A., Lemos, L., Rodrigues, E., Carvalho, A. N., Outeiro, T. F., Rodrigues, C. M. P., Gama, M. J., & Castro-Caldas, M. (2017). Nrf2 activation by tauroursodeoxycholic acid in experimental models of Parkinson's disease. *Experimental Neurology*, 295, 77–87. https://doi.org/10.1016/j.expneurol.2017.05.009

Ono, T., Imai, K., Kohno, H., Uchida, M., Takemoto, Y., Dhar, D. K., & Nagasue, N. (1998). Tauroursodeoxycholic acid protects cholestasis in rat reperfused livers (its roles in hepatic calcium mobilization). *Digestive Diseases and Sciences*, 43, 2201–2210. https://doi.org/10.1023/a:1026654219668

Rodrigues, C. M., Solá, S., Nan, Z., Castro, R. E., Ribeiro, P. S., Low, W. C., & Steer, C. J. (2003). Tauroursodeoxycholic acid reduces apoptosis and protects against neurological injury after acute hemorrhagic stroke in rats. *Proceedings of the National Academy of Sciences*, 100(10), 6087–6092. https://doi.org/10.1073/pnas.1031632100

Rolo, A. P., Teodoro, J. S., Palmeira, C. M., & Rolo, J. (2012). Tauroursodeoxycholic acid protects rat hepatocytes from mitochondrial and endoplasmic reticulum-induced apoptotic cell death. *Toxicology*, 302(1), 9–20.

Vingtdeux, V., Chandakkar, P., Zhao, H., d'Abramo, C., Davies, P., & Marambaud, P. (2010). Novel synthetic small-molecule activators of AMPK as enhancers of autophagy and amyloid-β peptide degradation. *FASEB Journal*, 24(1), 119–130.

Xie, B., Zhou, J., Shu, G., Liu, D. C., & Zhou, J. (2019). Tauroursodeoxycholic acid improves the motor ability of rats with Parkinson's disease through the AKT signaling pathway. *International Journal of Molecular Medicine*, 43(5), 2105–2112.

Xin, Y., Xu, L., Zhang, X., Yang, C., Wang, Q., & Xiong, X. (2021). Sirtuin 6 ameliorates alcohol-induced liver injury by reducing endoplasmic reticulum stress in mice. *Biochemical and Biophysical Research Communications*, 544, 44–51. https://doi.org/10.1016/j.bbrc.2021.01.061

Yoon, Y. M., Lee, J. H., Yun, S. P., Han, Y. S., Yun, C. W., Lee, H. J., Noh, H., Lee, S. J., Han, H. J., & Lee, S. H. (2016). Tauroursodeoxycholic acid reduces ER stress by regulating of Akt-dependent cellular prion protein. *Scientific Reports*, 6, 39838. https://doi.org/10.1038/srep39838

Zhang, L., Jiang, Y., Zhu, X., & Shi, J. (2017). Tauroursodeoxycholic acid inhibits endoplasmic reticulum stress and protects against cholestasis-induced liver fibrosis in rats. *Digestive Diseases and Sciences*, 62(9), 2453–2463.

Zhang, X., Wang, Y., Liang, Q., Li, W., Zhang, Y., & Zhao, L. (2014). Tauroursodeoxycholic acid protects retinal pigment epithelium from endoplasmic reticulum stress-induced apoptosis. *Molecular Vision*, 20, 139–148.

## Urolithin A

Andreux, P. A., Blanco-Bose, W., Ryu, D., Burdet, F., Ibberson, M., Aebischer, P., Auwerx, J., Singh, A., & Rinsch, C. (2019). The mitophagy activator urolithin A is safe and induces a molecular signature of improved mitochondrial and cellular health in humans. *Nature Metabolism*, 1(6), 595–603. https://doi.org/10.1038/s42255-019-0073-4

D'Amico, D., Andreux, P. A., Valdés, P., Singh, A., Rinsch, C., & Auwerx, J. (2021). Impact of the natural compound urolithin A on health, disease, and aging. *Trends in Molecular Medicine*, 27(7), 687–99. https://doi.org/10.1016/j.molmed.2021.04.009.

Freeman, N. S., & Turner, J. M. (2024). In the 'plant-based' era, patients with chronic kidney disease should focus on eating healthy. *Journal of Renal Nutrition*, 34(1), 4–10. https://doi.org/10.1053/j.jrn.2023.08.010

Liu, S., D'Amico, D., Shankland, E., Bhayana, S., Garcia, J. M., Aebischer, P., Rinsch, C., Singh, A., & Marcinek, D. J. (2022). Effect of urolithin A supplementation on muscle endurance and mitochondrial health in older adults: A randomized clinical trial. *JAMA Network Open*, 5(1), e2144279. https://doi.org/10.1001/jamanetworkopen.2021.44279

Luan, P., D'Amico, D., Andreux, P. A., Laurila, P.-P., Wohlwend, M., Li, H., de Lima, T. I., Place, N., Rinsch, C., Zanou, N., & Auwerx, J. (2021). Urolithin A improves muscle function by inducing mitophagy in muscular dystrophy. *Science Translational Medicine*, 13(588), eabb0319. https://doi.org/10.1126/scitranslmed.abb0319

Singh, A., D'Amico, D., Andreux, P. A., Dunngalvin, G., Kern, T., Blanco-Bose, W., Auwerx, J., Aebischer, P., & Rinsch, C. (2022). Direct supplementation with urolithin A overcomes limitations of dietary exposure and gut microbiome variability in healthy adults to achieve consistent levels across the population. *European Journal of Clinical Nutrition*, 76(2), 297–308. https://doi.org/10.1038/s41430-021-00950-1

Totiger, T. M., Srinivasan, S., Jala, V. R., Lamichhane, P., Dosch, A. R., Gaidarski, A. A., 3rd, Joshi, C., Rangappa, S., Castellanos, J., Vemula, P. K., Chen, X., Kwon, D., Kashikar, N., VanSaun, M., Merchant, N. B., & Nagathihalli, N. S. (2019). Urolithin A, a novel natural compound to target PI3K/AKT/mTOR pathway in pancreatic cancer. *Molecular Cancer Therapeutics*, 18(2), 301–311. https://doi.org/10.1158/1535-7163.MCT-18-0464

## Vitamin C

Fang, Y., Chen, B., Liu, Z., Gong, A. Y., Gunning, W. T., Ge, Y., Malhotra, D., Gohara, A. F., Dworkin, L. D., & Gong, R. (n.d.). Age-related GSK3β overexpression drives podocyte senescence and glomerular aging. *Journal of Clinical Investigation*, 132(4), e141848. https://doi.org/10.1172/JCI141848

Kaźmierczak-Barańska, J., Boguszewska, K., Adamus-Grabicka, A., & Karwowski, B. T. (2020). Two faces of vitamin C—antioxidative and pro-oxidative agent. *Nutrients*, 12(5), 1501. https://doi.org/10.3390/nu12051501

Li, Y. R., & Zhu, H. (2021). Vitamin C for sepsis intervention: From redox biochemistry to clinical medicine. *Molecular and Cellular Biochemistry*, 476(12), 4449–4460. https://doi.org/10.1007/s11010-021-04240-z

National Institutes of Health. (2021). *Vitamin C fact sheet for health professionals.* US Department of Health & Human Services Division of Program Coordination, Planning, and Strategic Initiatives. Retrieved November 5, 2023, from https://ods.od.nih.gov/factsheets/VitaminC-HealthProfessional

Tronci, L., Serreli, G., Piras, C., Frau, D. V., Dettori, T., Deiana, M., Murgia, F., Santoru, M. L., Spada, M., Leoni, V. P., Griffin, J. L., Vanni, R., Atzori, L., & Caria, P. (2021). Vitamin C cytotoxicity and its effects in redox homeostasis and energetic metabolism in papillary thyroid carcinoma cell lines. *Antioxidants (Basel, Switzerland)*, 10(5), 809. https://doi.org/10.3390/antiox10050809

## Vitamins D + K2

Anglin, R. E., Samaan, Z., Walter, S. D., & McDonald, S. D. (2013). Vitamin D deficiency and depression in adults: Systematic review and meta-analysis. *British Journal of Psychiatry*, 202(2), 100–107.

Asakura, H., Myouga, F., & Ontachi, Y. (2019). Molecular mechanisms of vitamin K2-dependent protection against oxidative stress-induced apoptosis in rodent and human hepatocytes. *International Journal of Molecular Sciences*, 20(17), 1–18.

Cannell, J. J., Hollis, B. W., Sorenson, M. B., Taft, T. N., & Anderson, J. J. (2009). Athletic performance and vitamin D. *Medicine and Science in Sports and Exercise*, 41(5), 1102–1110.

Gast, G. C., de Roos, N. M., Sluijs, I., Bots, M. L., Beulens, J. W., Geleijnse, J. M., Witteman, J. C., Grobbee, D. E., Peeters, P. H., & van der Schouw, Y. T. (2009). A high menaquinone intake reduces the incidence of coronary heart disease. *Nutrition, Metabolism, and Cardiovascular Diseases: NMCD*, 19(7), 504–510. https://doi.org/10.1016/j.numecd.2008.10.004

Geleijnse, J. M., Vermeer, C., Grobbee, D. E., Schurgers, L. J., Knapen, M. H., & van der Meer, I. M. (2004). Dietary intake of menaquinone is associated with a reduced risk of coronary heart disease: The Rotterdam Study. *Journal of Nutrition*, 134(11), 3100–3105.

Giudici, K. V., Costa, M. J., Gonçalves, A. C., & Ferreira, A. C. (2016). Vitamin D in the prevention and treatment of oxidative stress: A systematic review. *Journal of Nutritional Science and Vitaminology*, 62(2), 67–74.

Grant, W. B. (2017). Roles of solar UVB and vitamin D in reducing risk of cancer, heart disease, hypertension, diabetes and metabolic syndrome. *Dermato-Endocrinology*, 9(1), e1308609.

Holick, M. F. (2007). Vitamin D deficiency. *New England Journal of Medicine*, 357(3), 266–281.

Holick, M. F. (2011). Vitamin D: A D-lightful solution for health. *Journal of Investigative Medicine*, 59(6), 872–880.

Holick, M. F., Binkley, N. C., Bischoff-Ferrari, H. A., Gordon, C. M., Hanley, D. A., Heaney, R. P., Murad, M. H., Weaver, C. M., & Endocrine Society (2011). Evaluation, treatment, and prevention of vitamin D deficiency: an Endocrine Society clinical practice guideline. *Journal of Clinical Endocrinology and Metabolism*, 96(7), 1911–1930. https://doi.org/10.1210/jc.2011-0385

Ishida, Y., Zhao, Y., & Kitaoka, S. (2020). The roles of vitamin K in the regulation of oxidative stress and cellular redox state. *Antioxidants*, 9(9), 1–16.

Jain, S. K., & Micinski, D. (2013). Vitamin D upregulates glutamate cysteine ligase and glutathione reductase, and GSH formation, and decreases ROS and MCP-1 and IL-8 secretion in high-glucose exposed U937 monocytes. *Biochemical and Biophysical Research Communications*, 437(1), 7–11. https://doi.org/10.1016/j.bbrc.2013.06.004

Knapen, M. H., Drummen, N. E., Smit, E., Vermeer, C., & Theuwissen, E. (2013). Three-year low-dose menaquinone-7 supplementation helps decrease bone loss in healthy postmenopausal women. *Osteoporosis International*, 24(9), 2499–2507. https://doi.org/10.1007/s00198-013-2325-6

Knapen, M. H., Schurgers, L. J., & Vermeer, C. (2007). Vitamin K2 supplementation improves hip bone geometry and bone strength indices in postmenopausal women. *Osteoporosis International*, 18(7), 963–972.

Martineau, A. R., Jolliffe, D. A., Hooper, R. L., Greenberg, L., Aloia, J. F., Bergman, P., Dubnov-Raz, G., Esposito, S., Ganmaa, D., Ginde, A. A., Goodall, E. C., Grant, C. C., Griffiths, C. J., Janssens, W., Laaksi, I., Manaseki-Holland, S., Mauger, D., Murdoch, D. R., Neale, R., Rees, J. R., … Camargo, C. A. Jr. (2017). Vitamin D supplementation to prevent acute respiratory tract infections: systematic review and meta-analysis of individual participant data. *BMJ (Clinical Research Ed.)*, 356, i6583. https://doi.org/10.1136/bmj.i6583

Milani, P., Vassalle, C., & Maltinti, M. (2018). Vitamin D and oxidative stress: A review on evidence and mechanisms. *Reviews in Endocrine and Metabolic Disorders*, 19(3), 219–232.

Ross, A. C., Manson, J. E., Abrams, S. A., Aloia, J. F., Brannon, P. M., Clinton, S. K., Durazo-Arvizu, R. A., Gallagher, J. C., Gallo, R. L., Jones, G., Kovacs, C. S., Mayne, S. T., Rosen, C. J., & Shapses, S. A. (2011). The 2011 report on dietary reference intakes for calcium and vitamin D from the Institute of Medicine: What clinicians need to know. *Journal of Clinical Endocrinology and Metabolism*, 96(1), 53–58. https://doi.org/10.1210/jc.2010-2704

Schöttker, B., Jorde, R., Peasey, A., Thorand, B., Jansen, E. H., Groot, L.d, Streppel, M., Gardiner, J., Ordóñez-Mena, J. M., Perna, L., Wilsgaard, T., Rathmann, W., Feskens, E., Kampman, E., Siganos, G., Njølstad, I., Mathiesen, E. B., Kubínová, R., Pająk, A., Topor-Madry, R., … Consortium on Health and Ageing: Network of Cohorts in Europe and the United States (2014). Vitamin D and mortality: meta-analysis of individual participant data from a large consortium of cohort studies from Europe and the United States. *BMJ (Clinical Research Ed.)*, 348, g3656. https://doi.org/10.1136/bmj.g3656

Schurgers, L. J., Vermeer, C., & Knapen, M. H. (2002). Vitamin K supplementation: A simple way to improve cardiovascular health? *European Journal of Cardiovascular Prevention & Rehabilitation*, 9(4), 241–246.

Shea, M. K., Booth, S. L., Massaro, J. M., Jacques, P. F., D'Agostino, R. B. Sr., Dawson-Hughes, B., Ordovas, J. M., O'Donnell, C. J., Kathiresan, S., Keaney, J. F., Jr., Vasan, R. S., & Benjamin, E. J. (2008). Vitamin K and vitamin D status: Associations with inflammatory markers in the Framingham Offspring Study. *American Journal of Epidemiology*, 167(3), 313–320. https://doi.org/10.1093/aje/kwm306

Shea, M. K., & Holden, R. M. (2012). Vitamin K status and vascular calcification: Evidence from observational and clinical studies. *Advances in Nutrition*, 3(2), 158–165.

Shearer, M. J., Newman, P., & Metzger, M. (2014). The in vitro effects of vitamin K in enhancing osteoblasts and mineralization. *Oral Surgery, Oral Medicine, Oral Pathology and Oral Radiology*, 117(5), 683–691.

Theuwissen, E., Cranenburg, E. C., & Knapen, M. H. (2012). The role of vitamin K in soft-tissue calcification. *Advances in Nutrition*, 3(2), 166–173.

Tripkovic, L., Lambert, H., Hart, K., Smith, C. P., Bucca, G., Penson, S., Chope, G., Hyppönen, E., Berry, J., Vieth, R., & Lanham-New, S. (2012). Comparison of vitamin D2 and vitamin D3 supplementation in raising serum 25-hydroxyvitamin D status: A systematic review and meta-analysis. *American Journal of Clinical Nutrition*, 95(6), 1357–1364. https://doi.org/10.3945/ajcn.111.031070

Yoshida, M., Jacques, P. F., Meigs, J. B., Saltzman, E., Shea, M. K., Gundberg, C., Dawson-Hughes, B., Dallal, G., & Booth, S. L. (2008). Effect of vitamin K supplementation on insulin resistance in older men and women. *Diabetes Care*, 31(11), 2092–2096. https://doi.org/10.2337/dc08-1204

Zhu, D., Wu, J., Spee, C., Ryan, S. J., & Hinton, D. R. (2016). Vitamin K1 and vitamin K2 inhibit different stages of intracellular oxidative stress. *Experimental Eye Research*, 151, 122–127.

# INDEX

ascorbic acid (vitamin C), 6, 85–87
athletes, 110–112
autoimmune conditions, 27, 54

## B

bacteria
    and alcohol consumption, 36
    good/bad gut bacteria, 24, 51
    immune system vs., 26
    prebiotics for gut, 60–61
    and urolithin A production, 84
baking soda, 49, 50
balance
    of antioxidants, 11
    dietary, 24–25, 39, 93
    in exercise, 114
    of gut microbiome, xi, xii, 22–26
    in the immune system, 27–28
    redox. *See* redox balance
bands, resistance, 120–122
bases (vegetables and fruit), 24–26, 93, 94
B cells, 26–27, 30, 31
beta-hydroxybutyrate (BHB), 58
bicarbonate, 49–51
biking, 116–117
bile acids, 82
blood circulation, 102
blue zones diet, 90
body, the
    exercise for the whole, 103, 108–109
    imbalance in, 26
    intelligence of, 28
    lifestyle/supplements to serve, 39–40
    sleep and, 31
    supplementing natural processes
      in, 41
bone health
    bone loss, 109–110
    collagen peptides for, 54
    exercise for, 103, 108
    lithium orotate for, 64, 65
    L-leucine for, 67
    vitamins D and K2 for, 87
bovine colostrum, 51–52
brain, the
    cognition supplements, 44–45, 56, 60
    diet supporting, 96

    fasting for, 100
    gut–brain axis, 61, 82
    L-carnosine for, 61
    lithium for, 64–66
    L-theanine for, 67–68
    sleep and, 32, 129, 131
    trehalose for, 81
breast health, 74
breathing
    exercise and, 102
    sleep apnea and, 37–39
    through the mouth, 37–39
BReg cells, 29
butyrate, 25, 52–54

## C

caffeine, 133
calorie restriction, 99
cancer
    anticancer supplements, 46, 73, 78, 87
    breast cancer treatments, 74
    and circadian disruption, 36–37
    colorectal, 54
    intermittent fasting to prevent, 99
carbohydrates, 13, 91, 93
cardiovascular endurance, 103, 108, 113
carriers, mitochondrial electron, 18
cartilage, 54
catalase, 5, 8, 9–10, 14, 22
cell efficiency
    benefits of, xi
    and circadian disruption, 36–37
    diet for, 89–101
    exercise for, 101–129
    immune modulation and, 26–28
    redox and, 3–5
cell osmolarity, 47
cellular dysfunction, 2
cellular health
    and cell intelligence, 26
    and the circadian clock, 33
    and external stressors, 2
    via hydration, 47
    importance of understanding, viii
    lifestyle/supplements to serve, 39–40
    oxidative stress vs., 9–12
    via reduction and oxidation, 4

# ABOUT THE AUTHOR

William A. Seeds, MD, is a board-certified surgeon practicing medicine for over 30 years. He is Founder and Chairman of the International Peptide Society, Faculty Developer and Lecturer of the A4M Peptide Certification Program, and a leading peptide therapy researcher. He is Chief of Surgery and Orthopedic Residency Site Director for University Hospital, Conneaut, and Medical Director of Orthopedic Rehab and Sports Medicine at the Spire Institute, a USA Olympic training site. Dr. Seeds has been honored at the NFL Hall of Fame for his medical expertise and in treating professional athletes, and serves as Professional Medical Consultant for the NHL, MBL, NBA, and NBC's *Dancing with the Stars*.